SHINGLES

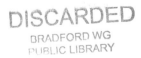

SHINGLES

New Hope for an Old Disease

Updated Edition

Mary-Ellen Siegel and Gray Williams

M. Evans
Lanham • New York • Boulder • Toronto • Plymouth, UK

Published by M. Evans
An imprint of The Rowman & Littlefield Publishing Group, Inc.
4501 Forbes Boulevard, Suite 200, Lanham, Maryland 20706
www.rlpgtrade.com

Estover Road, Plymouth PL6 7PY, United Kingdom

Distributed by NATIONAL BOOK NETWORK

Library of Congress Cataloging-in-Publication Data
Siegel, Mary-Ellen.
    Shingles : new hope for an old disease / Mary-Ellen Siegel and Gray
Williams. — Updated ed.
        p. cm.
    Includes index.
    First published under the title: Living with shingles, c1998.
    ISBN-13: 978-1-59077-137-2 (pbk. : alk. paper)
    ISBN-10: 1-59077-137-0 (pbk. : alk. paper)
    ISBN-13: 978-1-59077-141-9 (electronic)
    ISBN-10: 1-59077-141-9 (electronic)
    1. Shingles (Disease)—Popular works. I. Williams, Gray, 1932– II. Siegel,
Mary-Ellen. Living with shingles III. Title.
    RC147.H6S56 2008
    616.5'22—dc22
                                                                    2008007216

In loving memory of Hermine,

sister, friend, and staunchest ally.

M.E.S.

To my daughters, Julie, Meredith, and Dar,

who light my life.

G.W.

CONTENTS

CONTENTS

ACKNOWLEDGMENTS

Thank you to all those who support my professional endeavors: my family as well as my friends and colleagues in the Department of Community and Preventive Medicine (Social Work and Behavioral Sciences) at the Mount Sinai School of Medicine in New York. I am especially grateful to Drs. Helen Rehr, Gary Rosenberg, Susan Blumenfeld, and Penny Schwartz. —M.E.S.

Thanks to the many friends and relations who generously shared their own experiences with me, and helped me to gain a more personal perspective concerning this painful medical disorder. —G.W.

We greatly appreciate the many professionals who gave of their time and expertise to us to provide readers with the most up-to-date information:

Physicians: Brian Blakely, Christina Y. Chan, Seymour M. Cohen, Seymour Gendelman, Anne Gershon, Michael

A. Goldsmith, Joseph E. Herrara, Albert Lefkovits, Myron Levin, Jacqueline Lustgarten, Franco Muggia, Michael Rowbotham, Parag Sheth, and Charles B. Stacy.

Pharmacists: Michael Morelli and staff at Arrow Pharmacy in New York.

Thank you to the late Richard Perkin, founder of the VZV Research Foundation, and Louis Gary, the current chairman of the VZV Research Foundation, for their encouragement and for providing us with much useful information.

A special thank you to the late Mike Cohn, who brought us together on this project. And thank you to Rick Rinehart, editorial director of M. Evans.

FOREWORD

Until recently, physicians had little to offer patients suffering from a reactivation of the chickenpox virus, the condition called herpes zoster, more commonly known as shingles. In the past, physicians could only offer palliative therapy and home remedies. When antiviral drugs were introduced, the picture changed, and now more effective treatment is available.

Today physicians are seeing many more patients with shingles because there has been a growth in the population most vulnerable to developing this viral disease. This includes the aged, patients treated with radiation or chemotherapy for cancer, transplanted-organ recipients, people who are HIV positive, and anyone else whose immune system has been weakened by disease or treatment, or even excessive stress.

Physicians can now offer patients with herpes zoster effective therapy with antiviral agents if the condition is diagnosed early. If the painful condition known as post-herpetic neuralgia develops later, judicious use of carefully selected antidepressants, antiseizure medications, and palliatives can be helpful in ameliorating the resulting discomfort.

Anyone who suspects that he or she might have shingles should be examined promptly by a physician, since early diagnosis is crucial for effective therapy. The first seventy-two hours after symptoms appear offer a brief "window of opportunity" during which treatment can dramatically decrease the severity and duration of the disease. If a patient's primary physician is not experienced in treating shingles, there should be a prompt referral to a physician who is. Most family or internal medicine physicians and dermatologists are able to treat shingles effectively.

Most importantly, the recent introduction of the herpes zoster vaccine, approved by the FDA and recommended by the CDC for administration to patients over sixty, offers a safe and effective method of preventing shingles in patients whose age puts them at risk for developing this disease.

The authors of *Shingles* have researched their subject very carefully and have provided a great deal of information that should help make patients, their relatives, and their friends able to cope with this common illness. The authors stress that prompt treatment is important and that treatment is an art as well as a science. They offer hope for the present as well as the future in minimizing and even eradicating this condition once referred to as "the devil's grip."

Albert Lefkovits, MD
Associate Clinical Professor of Dermatology
Mount Sinai School of Medicine, New York
2008

1

WHAT IS SHINGLES?

Mark Singer is an avid gardener who spends much of his free time working in his yard. A year ago, when he was fifty-five, an itchy reddish rash appeared on the fingers of his left hand. At first he thought that he had once again come into contact with poison ivy. But he was annoyed that the usual remedies he used for poison ivy didn't work very well, and that the rash persisted longer than usual. Still, the itching wasn't serious enough to make him seek medical help. It was only because he had a regular checkup scheduled two weeks after the rash appeared that he mentioned it to his doctor.

The doctor examined the rash closely. "That's not poison ivy," he said. "I'm pretty sure you have shingles. Those little blisters are quite distinctive. A mild attack, fortunately. You're already getting over it."

Susan MacDonald was an active, seventy-six-year-old widow who had always enjoyed good health. One morning she got *up feeling slightly feverish, queasy in her stomach, and sore on the left side of her upper chest and back. Within a few hours a slight blotchy rash began to appear in the sore area. From friends who had suffered from shingles, she knew what the symptoms were. She called her doctor's office to report her suspicions and was given the first appointment for the following morning.*

By that time, some of the small bumps of her rash had swelled into blisters. "It's shingles, all right," her doctor told her. "We could have some tests run on fluid from those blisters to make sure, but it really isn't necessary. Besides, it's more important to start treatment right away. Fortunately your case appears to be only moderately severe."

As Fred Weintraub celebrated his eightieth birthday, he was thankful that he had no serious health problems other than mild arthritis in his hands and knees. One summer weekend, he noticed an odd, cramping feeling in his left chest, rather like a muscle spasm. Over the next two days, the cramping feeling became a burning pain which spread from his chest to his back. By the evening of the fourth day, a broad band of reddish rash covered the area. Thinking that this outbreak might be some form of skin disease, he went the next morning to a dermatologist who had treated him the year before for a severe rash from poison ivy. The doctor promptly diagnosed Fred's condition as shingles.

"I'm afraid you have a fairly severe case," he told Fred. "That broad band suggests more than one nerve is involved. And did you say that this is the fifth day since you first noticed the pain? We'll just have to see if we can bring this quickly under control."

AN OLD ENEMY, AND AN ENEMY OF THE OLD

The disease called **shingles** has been recognized since ancient times. Its most obvious symptoms—a blistered rash, accompanied by itching or burning pain—have long been well known. Also well known are several other basic facts: It mainly attacks older people, and the older they are the more severe the attack. It almost always affects just one side of the body, and it is limited to a specific area on that side. The most common of these areas is the middle of the trunk, and the second most common is the upper face.

Finally, and perhaps most importantly, the pain of shingles varies widely, but it can be agonizingly intense. Moreover, the pain may persist long after the rash has disappeared, a condition known as **post-herpetic neuralgia**.

The name shingles is somewhat misleading. The word is singular, not plural, and it has nothing to do with building materials. It is derived from the Latin word **cingulum**, which means "belt," and refers to the typical location of the rash, in a horizontal band around part of the chest or abdomen. Another word for shingles is **zoster**, a Greek word which also means "belt."

A DISORDER OF THE NERVES

Until the nineteenth century, shingles was considered a very mysterious disease. Why, for example, did the rash occur in only a limited area, and on only one side of the body? And what made it so painful? Fundamental discoveries about the nervous system, and the sensory nerves in particular, helped answer these questions.

It was discovered that the nerves that register sensations in the skin are laid out in symmetrical pairs, running from the base of the spine to the base of the skull. Each nerve of the pair extends from the skin to one side of the spinal column, where it connects with the nerves of the central nervous system, carrying sensations to the brain. Each nerve registers sensations from only a single body segment, called a **dermatome** (literally, a "skin slice"), and individual branches of the nerve may register sensations from only a part of the dermatome. That is why the area of shingles is limited: It almost always occurs within a single dermatome, or two or three adjacent ones, and it often occurs in only a part of a dermatome.

It was also discovered that the pain of shingles is neurogenic. Ordinarily, skin pain originates in the skin itself: Injury or irritation causes the skin cells to release chemical substances that in turn stimulate the nearby ends of pain-sensing nerves. Neurogenic pain, by contrast, is produced by damage or malfunction *within* the nerve cells—the **neurons**—that make up the nerves.

Neurogenic pain is characteristic of several conditions that are notorious for the suffering they cause. For example, **trigeminal neuralgia**, also known as tic douloureux, produces shocking, stabbing pain in the face, resulting from damage or irritation to the trigeminal nerve. **Causalgia** produces burning pain in the area of a nerve-damaging injury, such as a severe wound. **Stump pain** or **phantom limb pain** may follow the amputation of an arm or leg. The pain of shingles is similar in nature, and it can be equally agonizing.

DISCOVERING THE CAUSE

The basic cause of shingles was not identified until the early 1900s. Fluid from the blisters of shingles was found to contain particles of a virus—the same **varicella** virus that causes the familiar childhood disease of chickenpox. It has therefore come to be known as the **varicella zoster virus**, or **VZV** for short. It was also discovered that VZV produces the nerve damage underlying shingles, and that the virus tends to favor certain nerves: those serving the dermatomes of the trunk and head.

But it took several decades more to establish that shingles isn't caused by a new infection of VZV. Rather, the disease results from the reactivation of the same batch of the virus that earlier caused chickenpox. After a person's recovery from chickenpox, particles of the virus remain alive but dormant, stored in the **dorsal ganglia** of the sensory nerves. Ganglia (literally "knots") are enlarged portions of the nerve roots, which are located toward the back of the spinal cord (dorsal means "back") near the points where they connect with the central nerves. Usually many years after the chickenpox infection, the virus "wakes up" and starts to reproduce in the nerve cells.

Nerve cells—neurons—have a very unusual shape, compared with other cells. Extending from the main cell body, which contains the nucleus, is a long, thin tube called an **axon**, which contains only cell fluid, or **cytoplasm**. The cell bodies of the sensory neurons serving the skin are located in the dorsal ganglia, but their axons extend all the way out to the skin. The virus reproduces in the cell nucleus, and particles of it migrate through the cytoplasm of the axon. As they travel, they stimulate the neuron, producing neurogenic sensations of pain and itching. When they reach the skin, they are released from the branching ends (called **dendrites**) of the axon, producing the characteristic rash.

But why the long gap between chickenpox and shingles? The answer is the body's immune system. When you catch chickenpox, usually during childhood, your immune system learns to identify the virus and will quickly and effectively attack it whenever it invades again. As a result, once you recover, you will almost certainly never have chickenpox again. And although some virus particles "hide out" in dorsal ganglia, the immune system also prevents them from reproducing out of control. But as you grow older, particularly past the age of fifty or so, your immune system becomes steadily weaker. Eventually it may become incapable of identifying and controlling the virus any longer. The result: rapid viral reproduction, and shingles.

Further evidence of the crucial importance of the immune system in holding off shingles comes from a group of relatively young individuals who nonetheless develop the disease. These are the **immunosuppressed**—people who lack the protection of a normal immune system. They may be receiving drugs or radiation for cancer, or taking anti-inflammatory corticosteroids for lupus or arthritis. They may be suffering from blood diseases such as leukemia, lymphoma, or Hodgkin's disease. They may have been infected with **HIV**, the human immunovirus that causes **AIDS**. They may be taking drugs to prevent tissue rejection after an organ transplant. All these individuals, if they have ever had chickenpox, are at high risk for developing shingles. Moreover, the attacks are likely to be especially severe, and are more likely to result in serious complications.

AN EPIDEMIC OF THE OLD

Until the chickenpox vaccine came into use in the 1990s (see chapter 6), almost everyone contracted the disease, usually during childhood. Most adults still harbor the virus in the roots of our sensory nerves, and up to 20 percent—about one in five of us—will develop shingles at some point in our lives. About one million Americans come down with it each year. The chances of an attack begin to rise sharply after age fifty and steadily increase thereafter. If you haven't had shingles by the time you are eighty, your chances of developing it are about one in two.

For decades to come, shingles will continue to be an epidemic of the old. Moreover, as more of us live to a great age, more of us will have shingles. Not only will our immune systems become progressively weaker through natural aging, but also we are more likely to suffer from *other* health problems that harm the immune system. For example, we are more likely to develop, and to be treated for, cancer—chemotherapy and radiation are frequent triggers for shingles. Furthermore, the older we are when we come down with shingles, the more severe the attack is likely to be, and the more likely that it will lead to painful complications like post-herpetic neuralgia.

THE COURSE OF SHINGLES

For most people, shingles follows a typical course that lasts from three to five weeks. The course tends to be longer if the affected dermatome is on the trunk, shorter if it is on the face.

Sometimes the attack is triggered by a specific event. Your immune system might have been weakened by some other ailment, or by some drug you have taken. You might have experienced unusual physical stress, ranging from heavy exertion to extreme heat or cold. Or you might have faced serious emotional stress, from anxiety or grief, say, or a major life change. In many cases, however, the attack occurs without warning—"out of the blue."

The earliest symptoms, as the virus begins to reawaken and reproduce, may be so vague and unspecific as to be unrecognizable. You might have mild chills, a low fever, a dull headache, unusual fatigue, or a general feeling of being unwell (**malaise**). As the virus particles begin to travel down the neurons from the dorsal ganglion to the skin, you might experience sensations such as tingling, itching, or "creeping" of the skin in the affected area.

Even if you begin to experience the localized burning or stabbing pain typical of shingles, you still might not recognize it for what it is. The pain of early shingles has been mistaken for many other conditions, such as muscle strain, gallstones, appendicitis, or even a heart attack. But in two or three days or so, once the virus has reached the skin, the appearance of the distinctive rash should leave little or no doubt about the cause. Rarely—but only rarely—does shingles occur without this rash.

The rash typically begins with reddish patches of small bumps called **papules**. These soon turn into blisters called **vesicles**, which are filled with clear lymph fluid. The vesicles enlarge into **pustules**—blisters filled with cloudy pus, which is a mixture of lymph, white blood cells, and dead cell fragments. The pustules break open and then crust over and dry to scabs. The process takes place in successive, overlapping waves and usually lasts a week to ten days in all. The scabs may persist two weeks or more before they drop off.

Itching or pain may last until the skin heals, or even beyond. If it continues for several weeks or more, however, it is defined as post-herpetic neuralgia rather than shingles. That is, it is considered to be caused by lasting physical damage to the nerves rather than by irritation from an active virus.

Curiously enough, although the affected area may register powerful pain sensations, other sensations, such as touch or warmth, may be reduced. While the virus attack makes the pain-sensing nerves more sensitive, it tends to diminish the responsiveness of other sensory nerves. It apparently also diminishes the activity of certain nerve cells that inhibit the transmission of pain sensations to the central nervous system. This reduction of inhibition is believed to account, at least in part, for the intensity of neurogenic pain in general, and shingles pain in particular.

You might also experience muscle weakness, or even paralysis, in the affected area. Sometimes the reactivated virus spreads from the dorsal roots of the sensory nerves to the **ventral** (front) **roots** of the **motor nerves**, which control motion. Usually any such weakness or paralysis disappears when the virus attack subsides.

For most people, shingles is a temporary, self-limiting disorder. It may be very unpleasant, but usually it lasts no more than five weeks, never returns, and has no lasting consequences. But for a minority, the effects may linger. The most common and probably the most distressing of such possible complications is the continuing pain of post-herpetic neuralgia. Also, the surface of the affected skin may be permanently damaged, scarred, and partly numbed. Shingles of the upper face may infect the eye, risking at least partial loss of vision. Shingles in the area of the ear may lead to loss of hearing and paralysis of muscles in the face. In rare instances, the virus may spread to other parts of the body. In the lungs, it can cause dangerous pneumonia; in the head, life-threatening encephalitis.

WHAT YOU WILL FIND IN THE REST OF THIS BOOK

The following chapters of this book will provide you with further useful information about shingles and its complications, and about what can be done about them.

- *Chapter 2. The Varicella Zoster Virus.* Knowing more about the virus that causes chickenpox and shingles helps us understand the workings of these diseases and the ways that they are treated.
- *Chapter 3. How Shingles Is Treated.* Shingles can't be cured, but it can be controlled, mainly through drugs, but also with physical and psychological therapy.
- *Chapter 4. Post-herpetic Neuralgia.* The pain of shingles can continue long after the rash has healed, and special methods of treatment may be needed to deal with it.
- *Chapter 5. Other Complications of Shingles.* The virus can seriously damage vision or cause devastating infections in other organs, especially if it isn't treated promptly.

- *Chapter 6. Preventing Shingles: The Promise of Vaccines.* A vaccine to prevent chickenpox has already greatly reduced the incidence of this once almost universal disease. A new, much stronger version of the same vaccine shows promise in preventing shingles, or reducing its effects, for those who have already had chickenpox.

THE VARICELLA ZOSTER VIRUS

*S*usan MacDonald wondered how she had gotten shingles. *"Is it true," she asked her doctor, that shingles is caused by the same virus as chickenpox?"*

"Quite true," replied the doctor.

"Well, my little grandson comes over a lot, and he just had chickenpox. Could I have caught shingles from him?"

"No, the virus is your own, left over from the chickenpox you had when you were a child."

"Can I infect anyone else?"

"You can't give anybody shingles. But you might be able to give someone chickenpox, if that person hasn't already had it."

Susan was puzzled. "I'm not sure I understand," she said.

WHAT IS A VIRUS?

Chickenpox and shingles are both caused by the **varicella zoster virus**—varicella means chickenpox, and zoster means shingles. For simplicity, the name is shortened to VZV. Like all viruses, VZV is very small—thousands of virus particles, or **virions**, would fit into a typical human cell. And it is so simple in structure that it can barely be described as alive.

Each particle of a virus has just two basic parts. The core is composed of a single piece of either **DNA** or RNA, the long, chainlike molecules that carry the genetic code for reproduction. In VZV, the core is DNA, coiled up like thread on a spool. The other part of the virus is a coating of protein that surrounds and protects the core.

Although viruses are made up of the same materials as complete cells, they lack many essential cell components. They cannot reproduce on their own. Instead, they must invade cells and take over their genetic machinery, turning them into factories for more of the virus. The generated particles may then migrate from the host cell to invade other cells, spreading the infection.

Viruses are virtually everywhere around us, and we are exposed to them constantly. They can enter our bodies through the smallest cuts or other breaks in our skin, or through the mucous membranes that line many of our organs. Many of them are harmless to us—they can reproduce only in plants or other animals. But many others can cause human diseases, ranging from passing indispositions such as the common cold to dreadful scourges such as smallpox, polio, rabies, and yellow fever.

THE HERPESVIRUSES

VZV belongs to a family called the **herpesviruses**. Five of these are particularly important in causing human disease. In addition to VZV, they are

- *herpes simplex, type 1*, which causes oral herpes, or cold sores
- *herpes simplex, type 2*, which causes genital herpes
- *Epstein-Barr virus*, which causes mononucleosis
- *cytomegalovirus*, which causes a very common but often unrecognized disease of the same name, with usually mild, flulike symptoms

The herpesviruses share several significant traits, including the following:

- All of them require a human host. They can only reproduce in human cells.
- They are all very infectious. They are easily passed on from one human host to another.
- Once they invade a host, they never completely die out. They may become inactive, but they survive as long as the host does.
- Their effects upon the host are controlled by the host's immune system.

THE IMMUNE SYSTEM

The **immune system** is the body's main defense against outside invaders of all kinds. One of its main functions is to attack potentially harmful microorganisms—bacteria, funguses, and viruses—that make their way into the body. But it has others as well. In many individuals, for instance, the immune system triggers allergic reactions to certain substances they eat, breathe, or touch. The immune system also reacts against any foreign tissue introduced into the body, such as a transplanted organ, and it must be disarmed to keep a transplant from being rejected. And sometimes the immune system behaves abnormally, treating the body's own tissues as "foreign," and causing an autoimmune disease such as rheumatoid arthritis, multiple sclerosis, or lupus.

The immune system is based upon various kinds of white blood cells and chemical compounds they produce. The system is complex and carefully balanced, involving several different kinds of cells and several different processes. But it has two basic mechanisms. First, it attacks any substances that have been identified as foreign and either destroys them or makes them inactive. Second, it learns to recognize many specific foreign substances the first time they enter the body, and then remembers those substances so they can be attacked even faster and more effectively if they ever appear again.

YOUR IMMUNE SYSTEM AND VZV

Here's how your immune system interacts with VZV. The process is likely to start at some time during childhood, when someone who has chickenpox passes the virus on to you for the first time. Most often, the tiny particles of the virus are transmitted in invisible droplets of exhaled water vapor, which you unknowingly breathe in. The virus invades the mucus membranes of your nose and throat, multiplies quietly but rapidly, and spreads throughout your body. After two or three weeks of incubation, it produces its most conspicuous symptom, a reddish, itchy rash covering much of your skin.

Since this is the first invasion by the virus, your immune system doesn't recognize it and is relatively slow in mounting a counterattack. So you must endure a few days of chickenpox, while the immune system gains the upper hand. Your rash progresses from bumps to blisters, which break open and eventually scab over and heal.

Throughout this period, you are very contagious, expelling virus in your breath and shedding it in the fluid from your blisters. Any member of your household who hasn't already had chickenpox is extremely likely to catch it. That's why most people get the disease while they are still children.

By the time you recover, your immune system has not only killed off most of the virus, but has also learned to identify it for future reference. Whenever you are exposed to the virus again (and you probably will be, repeatedly), your immune system will attack it immediately and massively, preventing it from multiplying enough to cause any symptoms. You are now permanently immune to chickenpox.

Like other herpesviruses, the VZV in your body isn't completely dead. As explained in chapter 1, it retreats and hides out in the roots, or **ganglia**, of your sensory nerves, next to your spinal column. As long as your immune system remains strong and retains its "**immune memory**," the virus will remain there, contained and harmless.

But your immune system may become weakened by disease or medication. Or, over time, your immune memory for the virus may wane. The triggering circumstances aren't completely understood, but the virus may suddenly begin to reproduce in one or more of the sensory nerves, and then migrate back to the skin. You now have shingles.

Unlike chickenpox, the rash of shingles is localized within the area served by the affected nerve or nerves. The fluid in the rash blisters contains particles of virus, which are infectious. Thus, you can give chickenpox to someone who hasn't already had chickenpox and isn't immune to it. But you can't give shingles directly to anyone.

Not only is shingles more localized than chickenpox, but it may also be more severe. The nerve irritation is likely to produce not just annoying itching, but burning pain. The acute attack will also persist longer than chickenpox—weeks rather than days.

Unless your immune system is extremely weak, it will eventually regain control over the virus. Indeed, the acute attack should strengthen your immunity to the virus, so that you run only a slight risk of getting shingles again. Meanwhile, though, the virus may have caused serious damage to the affected sensory nerves. This damage is believed to be the chief cause of the persistent pain called **post-herpetic neuralgia**. It may last for weeks, months, even years, before finally subsiding.

VZV acts somewhat differently from the other herpesviruses. Whatever survives of **Epstein-Barr virus** and **cytomegalovirus** after the first infection is kept permanently under control by the immune system, and never again produces disease symptoms. By contrast, the cold sores caused by **herpes simplex type 1** and the genital herpes caused by **type 2** are notoriously recurrent. But because the immune system has learned to recognize the viruses and mobilize against them, later attacks are usually less severe than the first one.

ANTIBODIES (IMMUNOGLOBULINS)

Among the tools the immune system uses to fight infectious invaders are **antibodies**, also known as **im-**

munoglobulins. These are protein molecules that are produced by certain white blood cells to match specific invaders, such as a particular kind of virus. Whenever an antibody encounters the matching virus, it becomes attached to the virus particle, marking it for destruction by other immune-system cells.

Varicella zoster immune globulin (VZIG), a concentrate of antibodies to VZV, can be injected into individuals who have recently been exposed to chickenpox and need extra protection against the virus. These include those whose immune systems have been severely weakened by disease or medications. Also included are pregnant women, since chickenpox caught during certain stages of pregnancy can cause birth defects. VZIG can prevent or at least minimize the symptoms of chickenpox, so that it is less likely to lead to harmful complications.

One might expect that VZIG might also be helpful in controlling attacks of shingles and preventing postherpetic neuralgia. Alas, this treatment has been tried without success. Adding extra antibodies doesn't give the immune system enough strength to keep the virus from proliferating in the neurons. The only effective way to cut down virus reproduction is with **antiviral drugs**, which will be discussed in the next chapter.

VACCINES

The reason that diseases like smallpox, polio, and rabies are no longer such frightening threats to humanity is that effective **vaccines** have been developed against them.

The first and still the most famous of these is the smallpox vaccine, which provided a model for the others.

Through the ages, periodic smallpox epidemics killed or disfigured multitudes of people. In the eighteenth century, a physician named Edward Jenner noticed that people who caught a mild rash disease from handling infected cows never came down with smallpox. He collected fluid from the blisters of this cowpox and pricked it into the skin of people who had never had smallpox. They, too, proved to be permanently immune to smallpox. The serum he used was called a vaccine (from a Latin word for *cow*), and the process was named vaccination. Eventually, as we know, vaccination wiped out smallpox.

Jenner didn't know why the vaccine worked—only that it did. Cowpox and smallpox are in fact both caused by viruses, and the viruses are very similar. When the vaccine containing cowpox virus enters the body, the immune system learns to recognize the virus and to fight off any future infections of it. But the immune system also reacts the same way toward the smallpox virus, giving immunity to that disease as well.

The vaccines developed since then have been based upon the specific viruses themselves. The virus is either killed or seriously **attenuated** (weakened) so that it cannot multiply and cause disease. But when the vaccine containing it is introduced into the body, enough of its chemical structure remains for the immune system to identify it and form antibodies against it. The result is immunity to the disease, either temporary or permanent.

In 1995, a vaccine based upon an attenuated form of the varicella zoster virus was approved for use in this country. In the decade or so since then, it has proved enormously successful in preventing chickenpox. In 2006, a much stronger version of the same vaccine was approved for use in preventing shingles among those who had already had chickenpox. It shows promise in reducing the incidence of the disease, though not entirely eliminating the risk. Both vaccines are discussed in more detail in the last chapter of this book.

HOW SHINGLES
IS TREATED

M ark Singer's doctor was reassuring. "You're lucky," he said. "You're relatively young, your symptoms are mild, and your rash is already partly healed."

"Is there anything I should do about it at this stage?" Mark asked.

"Not unless the itching bothers you. You can use calamine lotion to relieve it."

"That's all?"

"That's all. There's no use in fighting the virus at this point. The rash will soon heal by itself, and you shouldn't have any more trouble."

Susan MacDonald's doctor was optimistic. "It's good you came in so promptly," she said. "The earlier we catch shingles, the better. We'll start you off right away with an antiviral."

"What does that do?" asked Susan.

"It's the one drug we can offer you," she replied, "that will actually attack the virus. Should stop it from reproducing in *your nerves. It won't immediately stop the rash and discomfort, but you'll hurt less, and, more important, you should recover faster."*

"I won't be taking antibiotics?"

"We're often asked that question," the doctor said. "Antibiotics are for bacterial infections. They don't affect viruses at all. I'd only prescribe an antibiotic if there was some sign of a secondary bacterial infection."

"Meanwhile, what can I do for these stabbing pains, and the itching?" Susan said.

"A variety of things. But you may have to experiment. Different things work better for different people. And again I have to warn you. Nothing is going to give you 100 percent relief until you're finally healed. In your case, though, I feel sure we can keep you fairly comfortable."

Fred Weintraub's dermatologist was frank. "You first felt changes in your skin five days ago, and the rash didn't appear until yesterday. That delay, along with your age and your serious symptoms, means that treatment may not work as well as we'd like. We'll start by attacking the virus infection, and making you as comfortable as possible. And then we'll have to see what should be done next. It's hard to predict."

THE ARSENAL AGAINST SHINGLES

Before so much was known about the cause and course of shingles, a lot of different treatments were tried to relieve it—most of them ineffective. Even now, no treatment provides a quick, complete cure. But modern medical science now offers a range of drugs and other treatments that are of demonstrated helpfulness.

These treatments fall into two main classes:

- *antiviral drugs*, which attack the virus that causes the disease, relieving the symptoms and hastening recovery.
- *palliative remedies*, which relieve the symptoms of the disease even if they don't affect its course. These include pain-relieving drugs, taken orally or applied topically to the skin, and techniques to reduce the psychological stress that often intensifies pain.

Treating the pain of shingles, like treating other forms of pain, is often best accomplished by using a combination of approaches: antiviral drugs, internal painkillers, topical medications, and techniques for managing stress.

ANTIVIRAL DRUGS

The **antiviral drugs** used to treat shingles all work in much the same way. They do not kill the virus, the way that **antibiotics** kill bacteria. But they do stop it from reproducing, thus limiting its power to do harm. Moreover, the drugs act selectively upon the virus, and have little or no effect on normal cells.

The process has three successive steps. First, when an antiviral drug is absorbed into an infected nerve cell, it provokes the virus there to produce an enzyme—a protein molecule that promotes a specific chemical reaction in other molecules. The second step is the reaction the enzyme promotes: the conversion of the drug molecule into a molecule that is similar to one of the building blocks of the viral DNA. Finally, as the virus tries to copy its DNA to form the cores of new particles, a converted drug molecule is substituted into each partial copy, so that the formation of the copy cannot be completed. In short, the parent virus can't have offspring—it isn't killed, but it can no longer reproduce.

That's why early treatment of shingles is so important. Antiviral drugs don't destroy the virus that has already invaded the nerve cells, nor can they repair any damage that has already been done. They can only prevent the virus from proliferating and causing even more damage. Thus, they can shorten the course of shingles and make its symptoms milder, but they cannot provide a quick or complete cure. And the more time the virus remains active before being checked, the less help the drugs can provide. So dosage should begin just as soon as a diagnosis of shingles can be made.

Unfortunately, that is easier said than done. The early symptoms of shingles are notoriously vague and unspecific, and are easily mistaken for something else. The only sure sign of shingles is its rash. And although the rash usually appears just a day or two after the tingling or pain, it may be delayed for several days, or even weeks. But you should go on "shingles alert" and seek the advice of your doctor if you experience the following:

- The tingling, itching, or pain occurs in a single area of your body.
- The sensation occurs on just one side of the midline, even though it may extend from the front around to the back.
- It grows progressively stronger and more constant.

- The pain feels sharp, stabbing, or burning (rather than, say, a dull ache).
- It seems to diminish somewhat when you lie down and relax.

And, of course, if you see any signs of a rash—even a few scattered bumps—in the affected area, you should get in touch with your doctor immediately.

Antiviral drugs are now considered essential for treating virtually anyone who has shingles, even though the attack may be relatively mild. Three of these drugs are the most widely used. The oldest is **acyclovir**, which has been in use for several years. Originally it was administered only by intravenous injection, and it is still employed that way in very serious cases. But now it is usually taken by mouth. The trade name for the pill form is Zovirax.

Zovirax isn't absorbed very efficiently from the digestive tract, so it requires five doses a day, taken every four to five hours except at night. More recently, two other drugs, **famciclovir** (trade name Famvir) and **valacyclovir** (Valtrex) have been developed, which retain more of their power when they are absorbed, and require only three doses a day. They work a little differently from acyclovir because they are **prodrugs**, which are chemically converted to active form during the absorption process

The course of treatment for all these drugs is a period of seven days, which experiments have shown to produce the best results.

Virtually all drugs may have negative side effects, but those of these three antiviral drugs are usually no more than annoying. The most common are headache and digestive-tract irritations—nausea, and either constipation or diarrhea. Less common, but occasional, is irritation of the kidneys. Famciclovir, in particular, may not be suitable for those who have kidney problems.

ORAL PAINKILLERS

Painkilling drugs range from mild, over-the-counter aspirin and acetaminophen to powerful corticosteroids and narcotics. They may not be capable of completely relieving shingles pain, but they can make it more tolerable, especially if used in combination with other methods. As mentioned earlier, they don't attack the underlying cause of shingles, only its symptoms. They fall into four main categories:

- *nonsteroidal anti-inflammatory drugs* (NSAIDs), such as aspirin and ibuprofen;
- *acetaminophen*, of which the best known form is Tylenol;
- *corticosteroids*, sometimes called simply steroids; and
- *narcotics*, also known as opioids.

Each of these types reduces pain in somewhat different ways.

NSAIDs

Nonsteroidal anti-inflammatory drugs have an awkward name, and they get it from what they aren't. That is, they aren't steroids. But they have one main effect in common with steroids: they relieve inflammation. Inflammation is a common reaction of cells to damage by injury or disease. The damaged cells release a variety of chemicals, some of which either stimulate pain-sensing neurons directly, or make them more sensitive to repeated stimulation (by lowering the pain threshold). Anti-inflammatory drugs block the production of one variety of these chemicals, the **prostaglandins**.

NSAIDs also have an effect that steroids don't. In ways not completely understood, they appear to relieve the perception of pain in the central nervous system—the spinal column and the brain.

So NSAIDs are doubly useful in treating shingles. They relieve the inflammation caused by the virus in nerve and skin cells, and they also reduce the sensation of pain, which in neurogenic conditions like shingles can be very intense.

By far the best known and most widely used NSAID is aspirin, technically known as **acetylsalicylic acid**, or **ASA**. The second best known is **ibuprofen**, familiar under such brand names as Advil and Motrin. Aspirin and ibuprofen are the only NSAIDs available over the counter. Stronger drugs, such as **naproxen** (Naprocyn), require a prescription.

NSAIDS have some potentially adverse side effects, especially when taken in large doses by older people. The most serious of these is irritation of the stomach lining, which may lead to ulcers and bleeding. The stomach contains powerful digestive acids, from which it is normally protected by a coating of mucus. The formation of mucus requires stimulation by prostaglandins, but NSAIDs hinder the production of prostaglandins. Lower levels of prostaglandins mean less mucus; less mucus means more acid irritation of the lining. Incidentally, the irritation can be intensified by alcohol. Even moderate drinking while taking NSAIDs may be risky.

One real danger is that the irritation may not be noticeable, and the resulting bleeding may become severe. Moreover, it may be compounded by another side effect. NSAIDs interfere with the activity of blood components called platelets, which are largely responsible for blood clotting. So, if the irritation does result in bleeding, the bleeding may be hard to stop. Aspirin has a particularly strong effect on blood clotting, and some doctors discourage its use for treating shingles, especially in large doses over an extended period.

The stomach irritation caused by NSAIDs can be somewhat reduced by taking forms that are covered with an **enteric** coating, which dissolves only after the tablet passes from the stomach to the small intestine. NSAIDs can also be taken with an antacid buffer to neutralize stomach acid, or the production of acid can be reduced with an antiulcer and antiheartburn drug such as Tagamet or Pepcid. But none of these expedients will completely remove the risk.

NSAIDs can cause allergic reactions in sensitive individuals. They may also interfere with normal central nervous system functions, especially in older people. Possible symptoms include headaches, dizziness, drowsiness, and mental confusion. Long-term NSAID use may hinder the ability of the kidneys to process wastes.

None of these adverse side effects are as likely to occur if NSAIDs are taken in modest doses for a short period of time. But the pain of shingles may require fairly strong dosages, and it may linger for weeks or even months. Bottom line: You and your doctor should closely monitor the use of these drugs, and it may be advisable to test occasionally for traces of blood in your stool.

Acetaminophen

Acetaminophen has overtaken aspirin in its popularity as an **analgesic**. It is probably best known as Tylenol, but there are many other formulations. It is also combined with aspirin, in such formulations as Excedrin Extra Strength.

Acetaminophen does not reduce inflammation. It apparently operates only upon the central nervous system, altering the perception of pain. It is comparable to aspirin as an analgesic, and many people prefer it because it has fewer adverse side effects. It doesn't irritate the stomach lining or hinder blood clotting, and it seldom causes allergic reactions. Large doses, however, may eventually damage the liver or kidneys.

Corticosteroids

Corticosteroids are natural hormones produced in the outer layer, or cortex, of the adrenal glands. Corticosteroid drugs are derived from the natural hormones, or resemble them chemically. For convenience, they are often simply called steroids, but they shouldn't be confused with anabolic steroids, used (and abused) by athletes to bulk up their muscles and improve their performance.

Corticosteroid drugs such as **prednisone** have powerful anti-inflammatory effects. Like NSAIDs, only more so, they hinder the formation of prostaglandins. But their use in treating shingles is somewhat controversial. They have several potentially harmful side effects. Like NSAIDs, for example, they trigger irritation, ulcers, and bleeding of the stomach lining. And they have other potentially harmful side effects that NSAIDs don't. Taken in large doses over an extended period, they raise the risks of elevated blood pressure (hypertension), bone weakening (osteoporosis), swelling of the ankles from fluid retention (edema), and diabetes.

Perhaps most important, corticosteroids tend to suppress the body's immune system. Thus, even though they may relieve the symptoms of shingles, they may at the same time reinforce an underlying cause of the disease. Nevertheless, many medical experts have concluded that the benefits of the drugs outweigh the potential drawbacks, especially when the symptoms are severe, or when there is a risk of serious complications, such as eye damage (see chapter 5). In any event, there is a general consensus that if corticosteroids are to be used in treating shingles, they should be used *only* in conjunction with antivirals.

Narcotics

The technical name for **narcotics** is **opioids**. Medical people prefer that term because it doesn't smack of lawbreaking and addiction. But the name is also more accurate, for it literally means "resembling opium." And indeed, the opioids are all closely related to that ancient pain remedy. They are either derived from it or chemically similar to it, and they relieve pain in the same way.

Opioids imitate and reinforce the action of chemicals that exist naturally in the central nervous system. Among the functions of these chemicals is to inhibit the transmission of pain sensations among the neurons. For the relief of severe, persistent pain, opioids are in a class by themselves; no other drugs are anywhere near as effective.

Opioids have other effects on the nervous system as well—effects that are both positive and negative.

- They affect the nerves that control the contractions of the intestines, slowing them down. This feature makes them very useful in controlling diarrhea, but it can also cause constipation.
- They can stimulate the central nervous system center that triggers nausea and vomiting.
- They reduce the activity of the cough center in the brain. A mild opioid like codeine makes a good cough remedy. But since coughing helps clear the air passages, suppressing it can complicate breathing disorders such as asthma or emphysema.
- They depress the central respiratory drive, reducing the rate and depth of breathing. This effect, too, may intensify breathing disorders, and an overdose can lead to respiratory arrest.
- They cause blood vessels to dilate, which makes them useful in treating heart attacks. But dilation also contributes to hypotension, an abrupt lowering of the blood pressure that can provoke fainting.
- They act as sedatives, generally reducing the activity of the central nervous system. Sedation reinforces pain relief, but it can also lead to drowsiness, impaired alertness, and loss of coordination.
- Finally, they affect parts of the brain associated with the emotions, diminishing anxiety and producing euphoria. Reducing anxiety helps relieve pain, but euphoria can contribute to dependence.

That's why many doctors are reluctant to prescribe opioids for any extended period, and why many patients are reluctant to take them, or feel guilty if they do. They fear that the use of any of these drugs will lead to addiction. The fear is mistaken. Opioids taken to relieve pain are very unlikely to produce euphoria, and virtually never lead to the compulsive craving of addiction. Although the process isn't well understood, opioids seem to be targeted toward the pain sensation, and their other effects on the nervous system are reduced. Furthermore, when opioids are administered under medical supervision, the doses can be controlled to minimize increased tolerance and dependence. People in pain shouldn't be denied these valuable drugs out of a baseless fear that they will become addicts.

Opioids are not prescribed for shingles unless the pain is fairly severe. They can be especially helpful when taken at bedtime, since they not only relieve pain but induce drowsiness. They are often combined with aspirin or acetaminophen. A mild form, such as **codeine**, **propoxyphene** (Darvon), or **tramadol** (Ultram—not an opioid, strictly speaking, but acting in much the same way), is usually enough to produce satisfactory relief. Stronger drugs, such as **meperidine** (Demerol) or **oxycodone** (Percocet, Percodan, OxyContin), are seldom needed for shingles. They are more widely prescribed to treat the severe pain of postherpetic neuralgia (see chapter 4).

TOPICAL MEDICATIONS

Many skin diseases are treated with **topical medications**—lotions, creams, ointments, and the like, applied directly to the skin. Their usefulness in relieving shingles is limited, however, because the pain of shingles results from damage to the sensory nerves, not just from irritation of the skin. Nonetheless, some of them appear to provide at least partial relief, especially when used with other forms of treatment.

Bathing

Technically, soap and water can't be considered a topical medication. But bathing regularly and keeping the inflamed area as clean as possible not only can have a soothing effect, but can also reduce the risk of bacterial infection, especially when the blisters begin to break open. When bathing or showering, keep the water temperature on the low side—hot water can intensify the itching and pain.

Wet Dressings and Compresses

A very simple but sometimes effective topical treatment is a wet cloth, applied as a dressing or compress to the inflamed area for ten minutes or so at a time, several times a day. The cloth may be soaked in plain cool or lukewarm water, or in a solution of salt or baking soda.

Anti-itch Medications (Antiprurients)

One of the symptoms of shingles is likely to be intense itching, and topical anti-itch medications (known formally as **antiprurients**) may give at least temporary relief. One of the most familiar is **calamine lotion**, based on zinc oxide and ferric oxide. It is sometimes supplemented with cooling agents such as menthol, phenol, or camphor. Topical anesthetics (see below) may provide relief from itching as well as pain.

Antiprurients that are *not* generally used for this purpose are the *topical* corticosteroids, although they are widely used for other kinds of itching. They tend to make the skin thinner and more fragile, and may make the broken blisters of shingles more susceptible to bacterial infection. Perhaps more important, clinical tests suggest that they offer relatively little relief from neurogenic pain. The same is true of another class of topical antiprurients, the antihistamines.

Topically Applied Aspirin

Some patients find that crushed aspirin tablets, mixed into an evaporating fluid carrier such as rubbing alcohol or witch hazel, or Vaseline Intensive Care, and then dabbed on shingles rash, offer at least temporary relief from pain. Some commercially available ointments also contain aspirin.

Topical Anesthetics

Topical anesthetics not only relieve pain, but also blunt all sensation by producing numbness. Their effects may not last very long, but they may nevertheless provide very welcome temporary relief. Among those used to treat shingles are **lidocaine, prilocaine**, and **pramoxine**. Lidocaine ointment and **EMLA** (an ointment containing a mixture of lidocaine and prilocaine) are commonly used for relatively mild or moderate pain. For more severe, enduring pain, such as that of post-herpetic neuralgia, an anesthetic patch, attached to the skin for several hours at a time, may be more effective (see chapter 4).

Topical Antibiotics and Antibacterials

As we've said before, antibiotics and other antibacterial drugs don't attack viruses. But if your doctor is concerned that your blisters might be infected by bacteria when they break open, you might be prescribed a topical antibiotic such as **bacitracin** or **Neosporin**, or an antibacterial such as **silver sulfadiazine**, for extra protection.

Incidentally, it is wise to let blisters open up by themselves. Breaking them open by pricking, scratching, or pinching increases the risk of infection, not to mention the risk of permanent scarring.

STRESS MANAGEMENT

Many people who have shingles notice that the pain may be triggered or intensified by psychological stress. The link between shingles pain and stress has important implications for treatment. Simple techniques for stress management can powerfully reinforce the effects of drugs and other medical agents.

Controlled Breathing

Often the best way to control psychological stress is physical relaxation. But achieving relaxation may require more than simply willing your body to relax, especially if you are in pain. Relaxation exercises, practiced until they become habitual, may help. One of the simplest is **controlled breathing**. Many people find it to be an "instant tranquilizer," which reduces physical tension and induces mental calm. It is also so unobtrusive that you can do it almost anywhere, anytime.

The controlled breathing exercise has four steps:

1. Either sit or lie down in a comfortable, relaxed position. If necessary, loosen your collar so there is no constriction around your neck.
2. Inhale slowly and deeply through your nose. Count up to five at one-second intervals. Between each count, think of a single word, such as *calm* or *peace*, to help free your mind of distracting or stressful thoughts.
3. Hold your breath for one second. Then exhale slowly through your mouth, counting backward from five to one, and silently repeat your chosen word. At the same time, let your chest and stomach muscles relax, and drop your shoulders.
4. Repeat this cycle at least three times, but continue for three to five minutes if you can. If the extra oxygen makes you feel light headed, alternate a few shallow breaths with the deep breaths.

Progressive Relaxation

Controlled breathing can be followed up with a more extended exercise called **progressive relaxation**. The way the exercise is usually performed, groups of muscles in specific parts of the body are successively tensed and relaxed, starting at the feet and ending at the head. However, this procedure may not be advisable if you have shingles. Tensing the muscles, particularly in the affected area, may in fact produce a pain attack. You might prefer a purely mental form of the exercise, in which you concentrate on each group of muscles in turn, and allow it to relax while forming an image in your mind of warmth and heaviness.

Either way, the sequence typically consists of the muscle groups in the following parts of the body:

- The toes of each foot
- Each foot as a whole
- The calf of each leg
- The thigh of each leg
- The buttocks
- The stomach
- The shoulders
- Each upper arm
- Each lower arm and hand
- The neck
- The face
- The forehead and top of the head

When the sequence is complete, the whole body should be allowed to relax while you form a mental image of sinking, going limp, and letting go. Like controlled breathing, this exercise should be practiced at least once a day until it becomes a habit. Some people find it especially helpful at bedtime, to help them fall asleep.

Meditation

While relaxation exercises help manage psychological stress by altering its physical expression, techniques of distraction work upon it directly. They are intended to relieve anxiety and the perception of pain by distracting the sufferer's attention away from them. Probably the best known and most ancient form of distraction is **meditation**.

Meditation has its roots in Asian religion and philosophy. Its traditional function is to separate the mind from the limits of ordinary reality and achieve inner peace. But it can also reduce stress and pain, and it can be performed easily, without any special training or grounding in either philosophy or religion. The technique requires only a quiet environment and repeated practice. Here are its basic steps:

1. Select a word or phrase that has pleasant, tranquil connotations for you. Always use the same word or phrase so that you will automatically associate it with the calming, restorative effect of meditation.
2. Either sit or lie down in a comfortable, relaxed position, and close your eyes.
3. Breathe slowly and naturally. Each time you exhale, repeat your chosen word.
4. Let your mind become otherwise empty and passive. If distracting thoughts intrude, try gently to disregard them.
5. Continue for at least ten minutes.

Once the procedure has become familiar and habitual, even a quiet environment may become unnecessary. Many people use meditation to create an island of tranquility in the midst of stressful surroundings.

Guided Imagery

Imagination can powerfully affect perception and feeling. The technique of **guided imagery** uses imagination to distract attention from stressful, unpleasant circumstances (such as pain), and to substitute a relaxing, agreeable environment in their place.

You begin by developing a mental image of a pleasant, tranquil scene—a favorite getaway in the mountains or at the beach, for example. You then try to direct your whole attention to that scene, immersing yourself in its details and experiencing it with all your senses. At least once a day, you set aside time to recall it, until you can do so easily at will. You can then use it to imagine yourself away from stress and the perception of pain. The technique has in fact been described as "taking a vacation from pain."

Sensory Substitution

Unlike other techniques of distraction, **sensory substitution** is aimed directly at the sensation of pain. Instead of trying to divert your attention entirely away from pain, you imagine that some other, nonpainful sensation has been substituted for it, such as coolness or mild prickling. This method may sound difficult, and it does require determination and practice. But some people find that it provides significant relief, particularly from pain in a specific, circumscribed area—shingles pain, for example.

OTHER FORMS OF TREATMENT

When the pain of shingles is especially severe, medications more commonly used for post-herpetic neuralgia, such as **antidepressants** and **anticonvulsants**, may be prescribed. These are described in more detail in the next chapter.

There are also a couple of techniques of treating shingles pain that don't quite fit into any of the categories we have discussed, but that have proved helpful to some patients.

Counterirritation

When you scratch an itch or vigorously rub a barked shin, you are making use of a natural, almost instinctive method of relieving irritation and pain: **counterirritation**. The mildly irritating sensations produced by scratching and rubbing are transmitted to the central nervous system, where they trigger reactions that diminish the sensations of itching and pain.

Some people find counterirritation methods useful in reducing the pain and itching of shingles. Incidentally, scratching is *not* one of them; breaking open the blisters raises the risk of bacterial infection. But for some people, just massaging the affected area with a towel brings at least partial and temporary relief. Some find it easier to get to sleep if they bind the area with an elastic sports bandage at bedtime. And some also are helped by **rubefacient** ("red-making") liniments and ointments containing **oil of wintergreen** or **menthol**. These dilate the blood vessels, causing the skin to flush and feel warm, but they also seem to work as counterirritants to the transmission of pain sensations.

TENS

A technique that is often used in the treatment of joint and muscle pain is also occasionally used to relieve shingles. It is called **transcutaneous electrical nerve stimulation**, or **TENS** for short. A portable machine produces mild pulses of electrical current, which pass through electrodes to the skin, provoking a tingling sensation (transcutaneous means across the skin).

Just how TENS relieves pain isn't known. Counterirritation may be involved. But it does appear to be helpful in some cases, and the low-energy electrical current is quite harmless.

CONCLUSION

Mark Singer's rash, as his doctor had predicted, subsided in about a week. Not only was he pleased that his attack was so mild, but he was also thankful that his chances of getting shingles again were much reduced. His doctor told him that only about one in twenty people who had shingles later went through another attack.

Susan Macdonald began taking antiviral medication the same day she saw her doctor. She also applied cool wet compresses to the affected area, and took a combination of codeine and acetaminophen at bedtime to help her sleep. In four days she felt considerably better, but at the insistence of her doctor continued to take the antiviral drug for the full seven days of the prescription. She also continued to find the wet compresses soothing, but soon switched from codeine and acetaminophen to plain acetaminophen and then to nothing at all. In three weeks, the rash was completely gone, and ten days after that, she no longer noticed any pain at all. She, too, was pleased to learn from her doctor that she was unlikely to suffer a recurrence.

After taking an antiviral drug for a week, Fred Weintraub didn't feel noticeably better. He took oxycodone and acetaminophen three times a day, and got some relief from applying an anesthetic ointment every few hours. Two weeks later, the rash began to heal, but the pain lingered on. He had trouble sleeping, and also suffered from loss of appetite.

His doctor shared Fred's disappointment. "I'm afraid you have post-herpetic neuralgia," he said.

Fortunately, most people recover completely from shingles within a few weeks, and antiviral drugs and other treatments help considerably to relieve its symptoms. Furthermore, once they have recovered, they have only about a one in twenty chance of suffering another attack in their lifetimes. Apparently the reactivation of the virus also strengthens the immune system to keep it in check.

But some people, especially those older than seventy-five, are not so lucky. The acute stage of the disease is likely to be more severe, and is more likely to be followed by the most unpleasant condition called post-herpetic neuralgia. We will discuss this condition and its treatment in the next chapter.

POST-HERPETIC
NEURALGIA

F red Weintraub was deeply disappointed and distressed by
the persistence of deep burning pain after the last of his
shingles rash disappeared. He was further upset by a new
and disturbing symptom. Any light, brushing touch upon the
skin in and around the shingles area produced spasms of
sharp, stabbing pain. It felt as if a cat were sharpening its
claws on his back and chest. He spent his days stripped to the
waist to avoid the friction of his clothes, and went to bed at
night without a pajama top or even a sheet over him.

Fred's dermatologist referred him to a neurologist with extensive experience treating post-herpetic neuralgia. "I want
you to try some different medications," the neurologist told
him. "As best as we can tell, post-herpetic neuralgia is a
rather different condition from shingles."

"Could have fooled me," Fred grumbled. "Feels like the
same thing, only worse."

"True," the doctor acknowledged. "But at this stage, other
kinds of treatment seem to be more helpful."

"Will they cure the pain?"

"For most people, they seem to cut the time it lasts, or at least make it more tolerable. But I don't want to offer any false promises. There's a lot we don't understand about this problem."

Estelle Freneaux had recently retired at seventy from a long and satisfying career as a medical librarian. She took pride in her knowledge concerning a wide variety of medical conditions—especially those likely to affect older people like herself. So, when she awoke one morning with a sharp pain that extended in a narrow band from her chest to her back, she suspected shingles, and immediately went to see her family physician. Although there was no rash, her doctor agreed that the symptoms suggested shingles, and prescribed an antiviral drug just in case.

A couple of days later, a few telltale bumps confirmed the diagnosis, but the antiviral drug, combined with an oral corticosteroid, apparently reduced the impact of the reawakened chickenpox virus. She needed only ibuprofen to control the pain, and in less than a month felt that she had almost completely recovered.

Then, even though the rash had disappeared, the pain became more intense. In another week or so, it was keeping her from sleeping, and she was no longer able to continue her normal activities. Her doctor regretfully diagnosed post-herpetic neuralgia.

"It's just not fair!" Estelle complained. "I did everything I was supposed to do, and I thought I was getting better. And now this!"

"I know how disappointed you must feel," replied her doctor sympathetically. "But post-herpetic neuralgia is unpredictable. Usually it hits people who have had severe shingles—

but not always. You seem to be one of the unlucky exceptions.
You'll just have to try the medications that seem to work best
against PHN, and hope for the best."

JUST WHEN YOU THOUGHT IT WAS OVER

After the rash of shingles has healed and the herpes
zoster virus is no longer active, you might expect the pain
to subside as well. For younger people with relatively
strong immune systems, that is indeed what happens. But
for a substantial number of older patients, the pain
doesn't end. It either persists or returns after a short interval, and it can be as bad as, or worse than, the original
attack. This is the complication of shingles known as **post-
herpetic neuralgia**.

There is no common, informal name for post-herpetic
neuralgia, other than the initials **PHN**. The medical name
may seem rather clumsy, but it is at least accurate. The
condition is indeed post-herpetic—it occurs only *after*
acute **herpes zoster** and is a direct consequence of it. And
the main symptom is neuralgia, literally "nerve pain,"
which arises mainly within the nerves themselves.

Estimates vary, but it is widely accepted that about
one person will suffer PHN out of every five who have
shingles. But the ratio varies enormously depending on
age. PHN is rare among shingles patients less than forty
years old, unless their immune systems are very weak.
But by age sixty, the risk of developing PHN after shingles rises to 40 or 50 percent. At age seventy, it reaches
70 percent or more. In short, the older you are when you
have shingles, the more likely you are to suffer PHN afterward.

It is hard to predict exactly who will get PHN, or how severe it will be, or how long it will last. It seems to occur more often among those whose shingles symptoms were relatively severe, and particularly among those who experienced noticeable pain before the shingles rash appeared. For some, the neuralgia is a mild annoyance; for others, an unrelenting, disabling agony. The majority recover within a few months. But some continue to have pain for a year or more, and, again, the percentage rises with age. For a small number—fortunately very small—the pain continues indefinitely.

SYMPTOMS

In general, the symptoms of PHN are similar to those of shingles:

- *Burning pain.* The most common symptom is a deep, burning pain, essentially the same as that of shingles, and typical of neurogenic pain in general.
- *Partial numbness.* As in shingles, the skin may be at least partly numb to external stimuli, such as heat, pressure, vibration, or even the prick of a pin. The numb area may extend outside the area of the shingles rash.
- *Allodynia.* **Allodynia** is a mysterious and very distressing symptom which is somewhat more typical of PHN than it is of shingles. The term comes from Greek words meaning "other" and "force." Allodynia is a spasm of stabbing pain, triggered by some other sensation that is not in itself painful. Often the sensation is a light, moving touch across the skin, of the

sort that can be caused by the friction of clothes or bedding, or by a light breeze. When the affected area is on the face, simple activities like brushing the teeth, shaving, or brushing the hair may provoke pain. Other potential triggers of allodynia include heat, cold, and sunlight. In some fashion, not well understood, these harmless sensations, transmitted through nerves that don't normally sense pain, somehow trigger the nerves in the pain pathways.

Like numbness, allodynia may occur in areas outside those of the shingles rash.

- *Other effects.* Perhaps even more than shingles, PHN can be physically and emotionally debilitating—simply because of its persistence. Common symptoms include insomnia, loss of appetite, apathy and social withdrawal, depression, and obsessive preoccupation with pain.

CAUSES

There is no disagreement about what causes shingles—it results from reactivation of the chickenpox virus. But there is no such consensus about what causes PHN.

On certain points, most experts do agree. Once the rash has healed, the virus is no longer active, and no longer the basic source of pain. PHN apparently arises from damage to the **sensory nerves**—not only the peripheral nerves that carry sensations from the skin to the spinal cord, but also the nerves within the spinal cord itself. And the affected nerves of the central nervous system are not only those that carry sensations through the spinal cord to the brain, but also those that control and modulate the strength of those sensations. But just how this damage is transformed into the pain and abnormal sensations of PHN is not at all clear. The mechanism of allodynia, in which pain-sensing and other sensory nerves somehow interact, is especially mystifying.

FORMS OF TREATMENT

Post-herpetic neuralgia is notoriously difficult to treat. Many of the drugs used to relieve shingles, such as antivirals, nonsteroidal anti-inflammatory drugs (NSAIDs), and oral corticosteroids, are ineffective against this disorder. No drug or other remedy offers more than partial relief, and none provides a complete cure. Moreover, individual response to different forms of treatment varies widely. Finding an effective approach must often be a process of trial and error.

Nonetheless, some methods do seem to be helpful, at least in achieving the two basic goals of treatment:

- reducing pain to at least tolerable levels
- shortening the course of the disease

These goals may seem disappointingly modest. Perhaps they are. But at the present point of medical progress, they are the best you can hope for. And they are more than you could have hoped for just a decade or so ago.

Four types of medications are especially supported by scientific evidence to be effective against PHN. They are the mainstays of treatment:

- *tricyclic antidepressants*, originally designed to treat psychological depression;

- *anticonvulsants*, designed to treat epileptic seizures;
- *narcotics*, technically called *opioids*, which block pain sensations; and
- *topical medications*, particularly anesthetic patches and ointments, and, to a lesser extent, topically applied aspirin and capsaicin.

Antidepressants

Impulses are passed from one neuron (nerve cell) to another by chemicals called **neurotransmitters**. Antidepressant drugs cause certain neurotransmitters to remain active for longer than they ordinarily would, thus strengthening the communication among the neurons they serve. **Antidepressants**, as the name indicates, are mainly used to relieve psychological depression. They influence the activity of neurotransmitters in the parts of the brain that process emotions.

But one type, known as **tricyclic antidepressants**, has also proved useful in the treatment of neurogenic pain—such as PHN. They apparently enhance the activity of those spinal nerves that hinder the transmission of pain impulses to the brain. In recent years, just as antiviral drugs have become leading tools in relieving shingles, so tricyclic antidepressants have become leading tools in relieving PHN.

The tricyclic antidepressants most widely recommended for treating PHN are **nortriptyline (Pamelor)** and **desipramine (Norpramin)**. As a rule, far lower doses of antidepressants are used in treating PHN than in treating depression. Most experts recommend that treatment begin promptly—when the shingles rash disappears but the pain persists. It may take days or even weeks for relief to become noticeable. And not all patients—about two in three at most—are significantly helped.

Antidepressants also affect other parts of the nervous system, producing side effects that are generally annoying rather than dangerous. Probably the most common of these is dryness of the mouth, caused by diminished salivation. It can be relieved with sprays of artificial saliva, but drinking more water or sucking on fruit drops may work about as well. Another common side effect is constipation, which can generally be relieved by bulk laxatives or stool softeners. Others include "cold" sweating, susceptibility to fainting, drowsiness, heart palpitations, and weight gain from increased appetite.

For one group, though, antidepressants can be dangerous. Those who suffer from heart disease are generally advised to avoid them, and a careful cardiac examination, including an electrocardiogram, is recommended for all patients before antidepressants are prescribed.

Anticonvulsants

While the most typical symptom of PHN is deep, burning pain, it may be accompanied by spasms of stabbing pain, either spontaneous, or triggered by nonpainful sensations (allodynia). These spasms are apparently caused by the uncontrolled, abnormal firing of pain-sensing neurons. They are therefore sometimes treated with anticonvulsant drugs—the drugs used to control the abnormal firing of brain cells that produces the convulsions of epilepsy. **Anticonvulsants** are also used in the treatment of another neurogenic pain disorder: **trigeminal neuralgia**, which causes pain in the face.

The anticonvulsant drugs now most commonly used to treat PHN are **gabapentin** (Neurontin) and **pregabalin** (Lyrica). Among their possible side effects are dizziness, drowsiness, blurred vision, and nausea. Along with tricyclic antidepressants, they are the most widely prescribed drugs for PHN.

Narcotics

Narcotics, technically known as **opioids**, tend to be utilized somewhat less than antidepressants and anticonvulsants, mainly because of their side effects (see chapter 3). Nonetheless they do relieve pain, promptly and significantly. They are often prescribed for occasional attacks of especially severe pain, or to supplement antidepressants and anticonvulsants, either when these drugs are just taking hold or when they fail to provide satisfactory relief.

Among the opioids, the one most prescribed for PHN is probably oxycodone (OxyContin, and combinations such as Percocet and Percodan), but there are several others. Codeine is generally considered too mild. On the other hand, tramadol (Ultram), a relatively mild opioid lookalike, shows considerable promise in treating PHN, just as it does for shingles.

If you take opioids over an extended period, as may be necessary to manage the pain of PHN, you may become physically dependent upon the drug. If so, when you no longer need it, you should taper off dosage gradually rather than abruptly, so as to avoid uncomfortable withdrawal symptoms. We must emphasize that such dependence is *not* addiction, and that you need not hesitate to take opioids to relieve pain.

Topical Medications

Some of the topical medications (lotions, ointments, etc.) that are used to treat shingles are also helpful in relieving PHN. They may provide only temporary and partial relief, but that relief can be very welcome. In general, they are easy to apply and have relatively few side effects.

In addition, there is one topical medication, capsaicin, that is specifically intended for treating PHN.

Topical Anesthetics

Topical anesthetics such as lidocaine, prilocaine, and pramoxine numb the tissues where they are applied. Their effects may last no more than a few hours, but they may provide significant relief when it particularly matters—at bedtime, for example, when you're trying to get to sleep.

Topical anesthetics are commonly mixed into sprays or ointments to be placed upon the painful areas of the skin. One preparation that has proved helpful to many patients is EMLA (eutectic mixture of local anesthetics), which is a cream containing both lidocaine and prilocaine.

A product designed to extend anesthetic relief is the lidocaine patch, sold under the brand name Lidoderm. Liquid lidocaine is absorbed into a feltlike compress and attached with adhesive to the affected skin for up to twelve hours at a time. Many people find it more effective than ointments or sprays, as well as more long lasting, in relieving the persistent pain of PHN. However, the patch itself, as well as the adhesive used to attach it, may irritate the skin, limiting its tolerability.

Incidentally, the lidocaine patch should only be placed over intact skin. That is, it can be used to treat PHN, but not the blistered skin of shingles. Also, as a general rule, the lidocaine patch shouldn't be used for shingles on the face, and it must be kept away from the eyes.

Topically Applied Aspirin

As we've said, aspirin taken internally seems to be of little or no help against PHN. But aspirin ointments, as well as crushed aspirin tablets mixed into an evaporating carrier such as rubbing alcohol, do seem to provide temporary relief for at least some patients.

Capsaicin

Capsaicin is the active ingredient that makes hot peppers hot. For medicinal use, pepper seeds are ground fine and mixed into an ointment, under such brand names as Zostrix and Capzacin. Applied to the skin, capsaicin produces a burning, stinging sensation, which may be followed by at least some reduction in sensitivity to pain. It is believed that capsaicin lowers the level of a neurotransmitter called substance P, which facilitates the transmission of pain impulses to the spinal nerves and brain.

But capsaicin doesn't work for everyone. A few authorities question whether it works at all. Like topical anesthetics, it must be applied very carefully (if at all) to the face, for it must be kept away from the eyes. And it has one other big drawback: It takes a good deal of getting used to. Just as you have to desensitize your mouth by re-peatedly eating mild peppery dishes before you can take on a really hot chili, so you have to apply capsaicin re-peatedly before the initial stinging sensation subsides. And many people just can't bear it for that long.

OTHER FORMS OF TREATMENT

A number of other approaches, ranging from acupunc-ture to nerve blocks, have been used in attempts to treat PHN. In general, though, they are not considered reliably effective against PHN, and for many patients they provide no meaningful relief at all.

Acupuncture

Acupuncture has a long tradition of use in treating pain, and some people maintain that it has helped them over-come PHN. But the hard, cold evidence of statistical stud-ies fails to support its effectiveness for this purpose.

Electrical Stimulation

Just why low-level pulses of electrical current should give relief from pain is unknown, but they are nonetheless sometimes effective. The simplest method for delivering such pulses is called **transcutaneous electrical nerve stimulation**, or **TENS** for short. It is used for shingles as well as PHN. Electrodes from a portable generator are at-tached to affected areas on the skin (transcutaneous means "across the skin"), provoking tingling sensations and for some users at least a measure of pain relief.

The devices used for **peripheral nerve stimulation** and **spinal cord stimulation** work similarly. They are implanted under the skin, either in the painful area or near the spine, and like TENS they can be turned on as needed to relieve pain. And like TENS they help only a minority of patients.

Nerve Blocks

Nerve blocks, which completely stop the transmission of impulses, are used infrequently but occasionally to treat post-herpetic pain. As a rule, they are only used as a last resort, when the pain is severe and long lasting, and other approaches have failed. They have many potentially serious side effects, and even the most radical of them—completely severing the nerves—offers only temporary relief.

There are two main types: blocks of sensory nerves, and blocks of sympathetic ganglia.

Sensory Nerve Blocks

The simplest nerve blocks are those produced by local **anesthetics**, injected near the spine in the area of the roots of the affected nerves. A relatively low concentration of anesthetic often relieves pain without provoking complete numbness. But the effect wears off within hours. Anesthetic blocks are used more often to treat especially severe shingles pain, but sometimes they are used to relieve PHN, in an effort to interrupt the pain cycle.

To achieve prolonged sensory blocks, the nerves must be severed by surgery, or destroyed with chemicals, cold, or heat. The procedure may be performed on nerve roots near the spinal column, on sections of the spinal cord, or even in parts of the brain. Needless to say, this is an extremely invasive approach. It produces complete numbness and often interferes with normal function in the affected parts of the body.

Even prolonged blocks may not provide permanent relief. After a few months, the nerves regenerate, or other nerves take over their work. But even temporary relief may be welcome, and the break in the pain cycle may lead to lasting pain reduction.

Sympathetic Nerve Blocks

The **sympathetic nervous system** is composed of nerves that control autonomic (literally "self-ruling") body functions, ranging from perspiration to blood pressure. The sympathetic nerves would seem to have nothing to do with the sensory nerves. But for some reason—perhaps because of certain neurotransmitters they generate—they can trigger or intensify pain sensations. Blocking them, either temporarily or for a prolonged period, can be particularly helpful in relieving neurogenic pain, such as PHN.

Sympathetic nerves come together in clusters, or **ganglia**, at certain points along each side of the spinal column. To relieve pain, a block is applied to the ganglion serving the affected part of the body. Like sensory nerve blocks, sympathetic blocks may be temporary or prolonged. Temporary blocks are achieved with a local anesthetic, prolonged blocks by chemical destruction of the nerves.

The side effects of sympathetic blocks tend to be less severe than those of sensory blocks, but some normal functions may be at least temporarily altered. Like sensory blocks, even prolonged sympathetic blocks do not give permanent relief.

PSYCHOLOGICAL APPROACHES

One of the most unfortunate aspects of persistent, or chronic, pain is what is called the **pain cycle**. Physical pain provokes psychological stress, which in turn intensifies the perception of pain, which leads to more stress, and so on. Furthermore, intense, unrelieved pain can do extensive psychological damage; it can, for example, lead or contribute to disabling depression and helpless invalidism. So psychological treatment can often be very helpful in breaking the pain cycle and coping with both physical and emotional distress. It cannot replace drugs in the relief of PHN, but can substantially reinforce them.

Stress Management

The simplest psychological approaches are basic techniques for managing stress, which can be undertaken by just about anyone. They are also useful in relieving shingles pain, and have been discussed in more detail in the preceding chapter.

They fall into two categories. One is composed of techniques for relieving psychological tension by means of physical relaxation. Such techniques include exercises in controlled breathing and progressive relaxation of muscle groups.

The second category is distraction. Its techniques are intended to relieve anxiety and pain perception by distracting the sufferer's attention away from them. The techniques include meditation, guided imagery, and sensory substitution.

Most of these techniques are also appropriate for treating shingles, and are described in chapter 3. But there are a few that are more commonly used to relieve PHN.

Biofeedback

Biofeedback is a technique that is most often used in treating chronic headaches, but some people have also found it helpful in relieving PHN. It might be described as mechanically assisted relaxation.

A biofeedback machine is essentially an amplifier of weak electrical signals, received from electrodes attached to the skin. The electrodes register physical signs of stress—slight muscle contractions, for example, or changing levels of skin temperature—as electrical impulses. The biofeedback amplifier then strengthens the impulses and makes them either visible (flashing lights or a moving dial) or audible (tones, beeps, or clicks). The higher the level of tension, the more pronounced are the generated impulses, and the stronger is the visible or audible output.

The biofeedback machine doesn't really *do* anything to you, except to inform you how your body is responding to stress. But apparently when you become more aware of stress, you are better able to control it, and better able to achieve relaxation. Through repeated biofeedback sessions, you may be able to retrain your nervous system to manage stress more successfully, breaking into the pain cycle.

Hypnosis

Hypnosis is an artificially induced state of consciousness—a trance—in which your attention becomes tightly focused, and you become strongly susceptible to suggestion. Suggestion under hypnosis can greatly alter perception—including the perception of pain.

Just as biofeedback can be used to reinforce physical relaxation, hypnotism can be used to reinforce psychological distraction. Hypnotic suggestion can be used to make a part of your body numb—as if it were injected with an anesthetic. It can also be used to reduce the pain experience, transforming it into some other sensation (sensory substitution), or diminishing its emotional impact. And the effects of suggestion during a hypnotic trance may persist after you emerge from the trance—a phenomenon called posthypnotic suggestion.

But hypnotism has one big limitation. Many people can't be hypnotized at all, and many more can't achieve a deep enough level of trance to make suggestion fully effective. Only a minority can be easily and deeply hypnotized. The usefulness of the technique in relieving pain is largely confined to that minority.

Cognitive Psychotherapy and Behavioral Therapy

If you are among the unfortunate few who suffer post-herpetic pain for a long period of time, you might find cognitive psychotherapy or behavioral therapy beneficial.

These forms of treatment may not directly relieve your pain, but they may help keep it from intensifying. Perhaps even more important, they may enable you to cope better with pain, so that it doesn't completely disable you.

Cognitive psychotherapy is a relatively recent offshoot of conventional psychotherapy, and shows particular promise in the treatment of chronic pain. Whereas conventional psychotherapy probes deeply into unconscious motivation through the analysis of dreams, early memories, and the like, cognitive psychotherapy concentrates on the here-and-now—the ideas and values that determine your reactions to pain. It aims to make you rethink these mental attitudes, so that instead of reinforcing your suffering, they will encourage coping and healing.

One technique of cognitive therapy is to encourage you to substitute positive "coping statements" for negative ones. For instance, instead of saying to yourself, "My pain is unbearable, and I can't go on suffering this way," you might be encouraged to say, "This pain is hard to take, but I've coped with it so far, and I'll be able to cope with it in the future."

Another type of psychological treatment for long-standing pain is **behavioral therapy**. Like cognitive psychotherapy, it concentrates upon the here-and-now—specifically, upon the effects pain has on your day-to-day behavior. It aims to reduce negative "pain behavior," such as wincing, grimacing, physical inactivity, withdrawal, or appeals for sympathy, and to replace the negative behavior with positive coping behavior. It is believed that these changes not only will enable you to live a more normal life, but may also make you perceive pain less intensely.

MULTIDISCIPLINARY PAIN CLINICS

Shingles is customarily treated by an individual physician—a family practitioner or a dermatologist. PHN is also sometimes treated by a neurologist. But if your suffering from PHN is especially severe or long lasting, you may find it helpful to seek treatment in a **pain clinic**. Such clinics, often associated with a teaching hospital or university medical school, offer comprehensive treatment using a team of experts that might include a neurologist, an anesthesiologist, a physical therapist, and a psychologist, among others. The team undertakes a thorough examination and diagnosis, and provides a systematic treatment plan—often involving several different forms of treatment at once.

The benefits of a pain clinic go beyond the collective expertise of the team members. The main goals are not only to reduce pain and speed your recovery, but also to help you restore and maintain normal function. The combination of physical and psychological approaches can help you cope with your condition and carry on with your life, even if you haven't yet completely recovered.

RECOVERY

Recovery from PHN is likely to be intermittent. Attacks of pain alternate with periods of relief, and the attacks gradually become shorter and less intense, while the pain-free periods become longer. The steady, burning, "background" pain may disappear either earlier or later than the spasms of allodynia. The whole process may extend over several months, and each recurrence of pain is likely to be both physically and emotionally distressing. But once the pattern of pain alternating with relief becomes established, you can at least be reassured that eventual recovery is on the way.

Fred Weintraub was prescribed both antidepressant and anticonvulsant drugs, plus a combination of oxycodone and acetaminophen to help control especially severe pain. But for two weeks he noticed little or no change in his condition. The steady burning pain continued, and the least touch might trigger clawing, stabbing spasms of allodynia.

He tried a capsaicin ointment the neurologist prescribed, but stopped using it after a couple of days—it produced so much pain of its own that he couldn't bear to continue. He got a little relief from the anesthetic ointment he had been using during the shingles attack, and even more from the anesthetic patches prescribed for him. He found that a controlled breathing exercise provided a little relief from the spasms of allodynia. He also found progressive relaxation helpful, especially when he was trying to get to sleep.

Overall, however, these remedies were very limited in their effects. Fred found himself constantly exhausted from both pain and lack of sleep, and he lost more than twelve pounds from an almost total loss of appetite. He didn't want to go out or see anyone, and became more and more depressed by his apparent lack of progress.

But then, a little more than three weeks after he started the course of antidepressant and anticonvulsant drugs, he began to experience short periods of relief from steady pain, and there were at least fewer attacks of stabbing pain. Three months after he had come down with shingles, he was noticeably improved. By six months, the burning pain had dis-

appeared, and wearing clothes was no longer an agony. But the attacks of stabbing allodynia took another three months to subside, and he still suffers a brief twinge every now and then. When this happens, he becomes terrified that the neuralgia may return, although his doctor assures him that this seldom happens.

Fred remains apprehensive, but thankful that his suffering didn't last any longer than it did. He has been hearing a lot of horror stories lately, about people his age whose pain has persisted for years. "I never dreamed," he says, "that shingles could make you so miserable."

Estelle Freneaux was also slow to find any relief from the antidepressant and anticonvulsant drugs her doctor prescribed for her. And the narcotic painkiller she was given left her so groggy and nauseated that she seldom took it.

Topical medications provided only limited help. Anesthetic patches provided some relief, but after a short time became so irritating to her skin that she stopped using them. She put up gamely with the stinging produced by capsaicin until it subsided, but then concluded that it was giving her little if any relief.

She tried an aspirin ointment and several sessions of TENS with no noticeable effect. She signed up for a course in meditation and found it somewhat helpful, especially at bedtime. But as the weeks went by, she became more and more depressed and preoccupied with her condition.

But about two months after PHN set in, she began to experience short, spontaneous periods of relief from pain. These respites gradually became longer and more frequent, and the pain also became less intense. But it took five months before she achieved recovery.

She still had trouble accepting the fact that she could suffer so severely after such a mild attack of shingles. "There's just no fixed course for this disease," her doctor consoled her.

"But all the medicines I took don't seem to have helped much, if at all," Estelle complained.

"We just can't be sure," her doctor replied. "For all we know, if you hadn't been treated so promptly, your PHN might even have been worse. Sometimes the pain goes on for years."

"I don't even want to think about it," said Estelle.

OTHER
COMPLICATIONS
OF SHINGLES

After retiring from her career as a freelance copy editor, Connie Persig remained an avid reader. When she was seventy-three, she experienced a severe, stabbing headache on one side of her forehead. She thought she was suffering from eyestrain and might need new glasses. So she went to see her optometrist for an eye test.

After testing her vision, the optometrist told her that there seemed to be no need for new glasses. "Mrs. Persig," he said, "your headache doesn't seem to come from eyestrain."

"What else could it be?" she asked.

"I'm not sure," he replied. "But how long have you had that rash at the tip of your nose?'"

"Rash?" she said. "I haven't noticed any rash. It must have just popped out."

"I don't want to worry you unnecessarily, but I think you should see your physician right away. An ophthalmologist, too. I think you may have shingles in that part of your face. And if you do, there's a risk that your eye will be involved."

"Is that serious?"

"It could be very serious. But you have a much better chance of heading off trouble if you get immediate treatment."

HERPES ZOSTER OPHTHALMICUS

The most common potential complication of shingles is post-herpetic neuralgia (see preceding chapter), but there are a number of others. The second most common is viral infection of the area of the face that includes the eye. Its formal name is **herpes zoster opthalmicus**. For convenience, it is shortened to **HZO**.

As we've explained before, shingles results from the reactivation of the chickenpox virus, usually in a single sensory nerve. Its distinctive rash then appears in the specific area of the skin (**dermatome**, or "skin slice") served by that nerve. HZO results from reactivation of the virus in one of the three branches of the **trigeminal** ("triplet") **nerve** that serves the side of the face. The trigeminal nerve is a **cranial nerve**, which connects to the brain stem within the skull (the cranium). The affected branch serves the area of the forehead, the nose, and (most important) the eye, so it is called the ophthalmic branch.

HZO is not uncommon. Although shingles occurs most often in the various dermatomes of the trunk, the dermatome of the ophthalmic branch of the trigeminal nerve is the most frequent *single* site of the disease. HZO is estimated to account for about 15 percent of all cases of shingles. And in over half of the cases of HZO, the virus directly affects the eye.

The risk factors for HZO are the same as those for shingles in general. The principal factor is advancing age and the weakened immune system that goes with it. Also at risk are those people whose immune systems have been weakened by diseases such as AIDS or by drugs such as those used in chemotherapy against cancer. It is weakened immunity that apparently allows the virus to "come out of hiding" in the nerve root and proliferate toward the skin.

Symptoms of HZO

As is true of shingles in general, the first signs of infection may be vague or even misleading. You might have a low fever, or suffer from nausea, or just feel vaguely "rotten." If you suffer from a burning or stabbing pain in one side of your head, you might think it is a migraine or the result of eyestrain, and even a physician might consider it a symptom of some other disease, such as **temporal arteritis** (inflammation of an artery in the temple) or **trigeminal neuralgia**. Only the appearance of the distinctive rash makes diagnosis certain.

A patch of rash near the tip of the nose, called **Hutchinson's sign**, is considered strong evidence that the eye will eventually be affected. The sign isn't entirely reliable, however. Some people who show Hutchinson's sign recover from HZO without any effects on the eye, and a few whose rash doesn't occur on the nose nonetheless suffer eye damage.

Potential Damage to the Eye

HZO is considered a particularly threatening form of shingles. The reason is simple: The eye is a relatively delicate organ, and is especially susceptible to damage. Moreover, the damage may be irreversible, and if it is severe, it may cause the diminishment or complete loss of a crucial function—vision.

Virtually any part of the eye may be affected by viral infection. The effects may become apparent early, during the period of acute infection, or they may be delayed weeks or even months after the rash has healed. Among the areas most commonly and most seriously affected are the following.

Eyelids

During the acute attack of HZO, the eyelids—particularly the upper one—often become red and swollen, to the extent that they may be nearly or completely shut. The upper lid may droop uncontrollably, a condition called **ptosis**. These conditions usually disappear when the acute attack ends, but if the inflammation is severe, the lids may become permanently damaged. Some of the lashes may be lost, and the lids may not close properly.

Conjunctiva and Sclera

The conjunctiva is a thin, transparent mucous membrane which covers and protects the white of the eye. The **sclera** includes the white of the eye, and other outer layers of the eyeball. The invading virus may cause inflammation of either or both of these tissues—conditions called **conjunctivitis** and scleritis. The inflammations may be very painful, but usually subside without causing permanent damage.

Cornea

The **cornea** is a transparent window of tissue in the front of the eye, through which light must pass on its way to the pupil. If the cornea is damaged, the light may be distorted or at least partly blocked so that no clear image can be received.

Inflammation of the cornea, or **keratitis**, is one of the most frequent consequences of HZO, and it can be very serious. In most instances it is painful but only temporary. Sometimes it leads, either directly or by secondary bacterial infection, to permanent ulceration or scarring that impairs vision.

Uvea

The **uvea** (from a Latin word meaning "grape") is a group of connected tissues within the eyeball. It has three main elements:

- The **iris** is a doughnut-shaped ring that controls the amount of light passing through the pupil. It adjusts to different light levels, dilating in dim twilight and contracting in the bright glare of day. The iris also contains the pigment that gives the eye its distinctive color.
- The **ciliary body** is a muscular ring outside the iris. It is connected by threadlike extensions (cilia) to the transparent lens that focuses light into a sharp image on the **retina** at the back of the eye. The ciliary body controls the thickness of the lens so that it can focus differently on close and distant objects. The ciliary body also produces, or secretes, a clear, watery fluid into the space between the lens and the cornea.

- The **choroid** is the inner lining of the eyeball. The retina is attached to the rear portion of it.

Inflammation of any or all of these elements, called uveitis, may cause lasting damage, not only to the uvea, but also to other parts of the eye.

For example, inflammation of the iris (iritis) can lead to the vision-threatening disorder called **glaucoma**. Between the cornea and the lens are two interconnected chambers, separated by the iris. The watery fluid produced by the ciliary body flows steadily into one of the chambers, passes through the pupil, and is just as steadily drained out of the other one, so that the amount in the chambers remains steady. Severe iritis may cause scarring that blocks the drainage channels, and accumulating fluid in the chambers may exert enough pressure through the lens to raise the pressure in the jellylike fluid in the rest of the eyeball. This pressure may in turn damage the **optic nerve**, which carries visual information from the retina to the brain. The eventual result may be limited, "tunnel" vision, or, in extreme cases, blindness in that eye.

Lens

Inflammation around the lens of the eye may produce a cloudy area, or **cataract**, within it. A small cataract may have no noticeable impact, but an extensive one can dim or even block vision.

Retina

Viral inflammation of the retina may cause a condition called **acute retinal necrosis**, which in turn can lead to separation, or detachment, of the retina from the lining of the eyeball. A detached retina requires immediate treatment to prevent lasting harm to vision.

Muscles Controlling Eye Movement

A network of muscles around each eye controls its movement and enables the eyes to work together as a pair. Inflammation from HZO may damage the motor nerves controlling these muscles, so that the affected eye can no longer coordinate properly with the normal one. The result may be blurry or double vision, which is usually only temporary.

Treatment of HZO

Because the possible effects of HZO can be so devastating, it is especially important to get treatment just as soon as the diagnosis becomes clear. In general, HZO is treated with the same methods used for other forms of shingles (see chapter 3). An ophthalmologist should be part of the professional team, to monitor for such adverse effects as glaucoma.

Incidentally, two medications should be avoided in treating post-herpetic neuralgia (PHN) on the head: the lidocaine patch and capsaicin.

Antiviral Drugs

The most promising tools for treating HZO are the antiviral drugs—acyclovir, famciclovir, and valacyclovir—used for other forms of shingles. The sooner they are taken, the better. If more than three days (seventy-two hours) go by after the outbreak of the rash, the chances are that the drugs won't be fully effective. If the inflammation is especially severe, it may be advisable to have acyclovir administered intravenously. This may be a great nuisance, but the stakes are high.

Antiviral drugs are best taken internally. Topical antivirals—drops and ointments—are available, but there is general agreement that they do little to relieve HZO, since the damage to the eye is caused by inflammation, rather than by the viral infection. There is virtually universal agreement that the topicals are no substitute for the pills or injections.

Analgesics

Analgesics (painkillers)—especially nonsteroidal anti-inflammatory drugs (NSAIDs) such as aspirin and ibuprofen—can be useful in reducing both the pain and the inflammation of HZO. Stronger drugs, such as narcotics (opioids), are seldom necessary.

Corticosteroids

The use of corticosteroid drugs for treating HZO is controversial, but less so than for treating shingles at other sites. Because the consequences of severe eye inflammation are so potentially devastating, many ophthalmologists feel that the benefits of corticosteroids outweigh their risks, except in special instances, such as in the case of severely immunosuppressed patients, or those also suffering from herpes simplex infections. Corticosteroids can be applied topically or taken internally.

Lubricating Drops

Keeping the surface of the eye moist with lubricating drops or artificial tears can reduce irritation and promote healing.

Topical Antibiotics

Some ophthalmologists recommend applying topical antibiotic drops or ointments to the eyes to reduce the risk of secondary bacterial infection in the inflamed eyelids, conjunctiva, sclera, and cornea.

Treatment for the Consequences of HZO

Many of the adverse effects on the eye can be treated, if not completely remedied, with techniques that range from drugs to surgery.

Surgery

Damaged eyelids can often be repaired with plastic surgery. Damaged conjunctival membranes usually repair themselves, but if necessary they can sometimes be repaired surgically, or even replaced with transplants. Replacement with a human transplant is the standard treatment for a badly damaged cornea. A lens with a vision-impairing cataract is now customarily replaced with an artificial substitute.

Treatment for Glaucoma

One of the main reasons for including an ophthalmologist in the treatment team is to watch for signs of glaucoma—particularly increased pressure within the eye. Glaucoma is mainly treated with drugs, many applied as eyedrops. Some of these drugs decrease the production of watery fluid in the chambers between the lens and the cornea. Others help to keep the drainage channels open. In severe cases, surgery may eventually become necessary to provide drainage.

RAMSAY HUNT SYNDROME

The seventh pair of cranial nerves are called the **facial nerves**. They are composite nerves, which have both sensory and motor branches. Their sensory branches register sensations in the area of the ear, and also the sense of taste in the forward part of the tongue. Their motor branches control the muscles of facial expression.

Shingles in one of the facial nerves is uncommon but not rare, and is likely to involve other nearby nerves as well, such as the pain-sensing trigeminal nerve, and the **acoustic nerve**, which registers sensations of hearing and balance in the inner ear. The result is known as **Ramsay Hunt syndrome**, and its typical symptoms include the following:

- Severe earache
- Shingles rash on and near the ear, and in the ear canal
- Loss of taste in part of the tongue
- Paralysis of the facial muscles
- Partial or complete loss of hearing

- Inner ear disturbances, resulting in dizziness (vertigo) or nausea

Some of these symptoms, such as the rash, ear pain, dizziness and nausea, and partial loss of taste are temporary, and pass off with the acute infection. But the facial paralysis and hearing loss may linger for some time, and, in rare instances, may last indefinitely.

Like other forms of shingles, Ramsay Hunt syndrome is treated with antiviral drugs, anti-inflammatory and narcotic analgesics, and sometimes corticosteroids. The antianxiety drug **diazepam** (Valium) may be prescribed to control dizziness. If facial paralysis persists after the acute stage, it can sometimes be relieved by surgically enlarging the channel where the nerve passes through the skull.

SCARRING

A common but relatively less serious complication of shingles is imperfect healing of the affected skin. This is especially likely to occur when the skin is infected by bacteria as well as the virus. Instead of normal skin tissue, fibrous scar tissue forms. The scarred skin surface is abnormally smooth, and is often tight and slightly shiny. At first it may be discolored, and in time it usually turns a pale, silvery color. Furthermore, the area tends to lack some sensory nerve endings, so it may be at least partially numb.

Scarring is usually no more than a nuisance, but it can be unsightly or even disfiguring on the face. Sometimes the damage can be concealed with cosmetics or repaired by plastic surgery.

RECURRENCE

Usually if you have shingles once, you won't get it again for the rest of your life. But about one in twenty people who have shingles do suffer one or more later attacks. About half of these attacks recur in the same dermatome as before; the other half turn up elsewhere. Most affected individuals are severely immunosuppressed—their immune systems are greatly weakened by a disease such as AIDS, by drugs used to prevent rejection of an organ transplant, or by radiation or chemotherapy for cancer. Some are susceptible due to extreme old age. Recurrences are treated with the same techniques as those used for primary attacks.

Whether the new shingles vaccine (see chapter 6) can prevent recurrence has not yet been established.

DISSEMINATION

Shingles is almost always confined to a single dermatome, or at most to two or three adjacent ones. Only in rare instances does the disease spread into other parts of the body, producing a rash elsewhere on the skin, or affecting other organs. Disseminated shingles is almost entirely confined to the severely immunosuppressed.

The spread of the virus to the internal organs of the body can be very dangerous. Two potential complications are likely to be especially serious: pneumonia and encephalitis.

Pneumonia

When a person first catches chickenpox, the varicella zoster virus spreads throughout the body, including the lungs. Children seldom suffer any ill effects, but adolescents and adults, who tend to be more seriously affected by chickenpox, occasionally suffer inflammation of the lungs, or viral **pneumonia**. The same disorder sometimes follows disseminated shingles. Small air sacs of the lungs become inflamed and full of mucus and fluid, impairing the absorption of vital oxygen into the blood. In very severe instances, pneumonia can be life threatening.

The main treatment for viral pneumonia is antiviral drugs, as it is for all forms of shingles. Anti-inflammatory analgesics are used to reduce pain and fever. Since there is a high risk for secondary infection by bacteria, antibiotics may be given to head it off.

Encephalitis

Encephalitis is an inflammation of the brain and its surrounding membranes. It is an uncommon disease, usually caused by some kind of viral infection. Like viral pneumonia, it is an occasional complication of both late-onset chickenpox and shingles.

When the virus inflames the brain and its membranes, it can cause direct damage to the cells. Moreover, when white blood cells of the immune system accumulate to fight the invaders, the tissues swell, and since there is no extra space within the skull for the swelling to expand into, pressure builds up, destroying brain cells or causing bleeding into the brain. The results may be brain damage or even death.

In the treatment of encephalitis, antiviral drugs are used to diminish the viral infection. Corticosteroids may be used to reduce inflammation and swelling. Anticonvulsant drugs may be needed to prevent or treat seizures.

Anti-inflammatory analgesics may help relieve fever and pain.

Connie Persig called her family physician from the optometrist's office, and received immediate references to a dermatologist and an ophthalmologist. When they heard that she might have shingles near the eye, they both gave her appointments right away. The dermatologist started her on antiviral drugs that day. The ophthalmologist performed a thorough examination, including measurement of the pressure within the eye, which could reveal glaucoma. She prescribed drops to relieve inflammation, and scheduled regular follow-up appointments.

For a few days, Connie felt even worse. The rash spread to her upper cheek and forehead, and the burning pain became more severe. Her eyelids became swollen almost shut, and the eye itself became bloodshot and felt as if it had a cinder stuck in it. A combination of aspirin and codeine seemed to provide some relief and helped her sleep. So did cool, wet compresses and the anti-inflammatory eyedrops.

After a week, however, she began to notice a slight improvement, and then felt a little better every day. The ophthalmologist reassured her that the infection apparently hadn't spread beyond the conjunctiva, and that there were no signs of glaucoma. The swelling of the eyelids subsided, and by three weeks most of the rash was crusted over.

By five weeks, the rash was healed over, leaving no evident scars. The pain continued for about three weeks longer, and then was interrupted by pain-free intervals that became progressively longer and more frequent. By three months, she was almost entirely recovered, but continued to suffer occasional twinges, especially when she was tired or stressed. She returned periodically to be examined by the ophthalmologist, who had warned her that eye complications might crop up after her shingles disappeared. So far, though, she has had no problems

A CAUSE FOR CAUTIOUS CONCERN

You might find this account of the possible complications of shingles rather alarming. Please be reassured. First of all, the only really common complication is post-herpetic neuralgia, and, in most instances, even that painful condition resolves itself within a few months. Herpes zoster opthalmicus (HZO) is fairly common, but only a small minority of those affected suffer serious damage to the eye. Skin scarring is not uncommon, but is usually not serious. Recurrence of shingles affects a relatively small proportion of those affected—about 5 percent.

Other potential complications range from uncommon to rare. Ramsay Hunt syndrome is very uncommon, and lasting facial paralysis or hearing loss even more so. Disseminated shingles occurs only among a small number of those whose immune systems are severely weakened, and pneumonia and encephalitis are rare even within that group.

Furthermore, many of the potential consequences—even the serious ones—can be successfully treated so that the damage isn't permanent. And, finally, very, very few of these conditions are at all life threatening.

It should be plain by now that the best way you can avoid such complications, or at least diminish their impact, is to obtain antiviral treatment promptly—just as soon as shingles is diagnosed. Complications are more likely to occur when the shingles attack itself is severe and long lasting. Antiviral drugs greatly improve your chances of quick and easy recovery, but only if they are taken soon after the virus begins to reactivate. So if you have even vague symptoms that might signal the beginning of shingles (see chapter 3), don't hesitate to seek professional help.

PREVENTING SHINGLES: THE PROMISE OF VACCINES

Catherine O'Fallon took her baby daughter to the pediatrician for a twelve-month checkup. "Now is the time," the doctor told her, "for Sheila to have her MMRV immunization. That's for measles, mumps, rubella, and varicella—chickenpox."

"I'm a little surprised that chickenpox is lumped in with the others, said Mrs. O'Fallon. "When I was growing up, chickenpox was something we were supposed to catch—while we were young—so we wouldn't get it more seriously later on."

"Yes," replied the doctor, "that used to be the prevailing wisdom."

"And we thought it was particularly important for girls to get it over with, so we wouldn't come down with it during pregnancy."

"Right. Before the vaccine came along, that seemed the wisest course. But now that we've found immunization gives long-lasting protection, our thinking has changed. You see, even small children sometimes have serious complications *from chickenpox. It's better if they never get it at all. And there's another advantage as well."*

"What's that?"

"Shingles. If Sheila's immune to chickenpox without ever having the disease, she may never have shingles."

THE PROSPECTS FOR PREVENTION

Never have shingles? A very attractive prospect. Until fairly recently, it didn't seem possible. Most people—well over 90 percent of the population—would catch chickenpox, usually in childhood. Then, about one in five would later come down with shingles. Furthermore, as life expectancy increased, it appeared that the incidence of shingles could only rise as well. But two related breakthroughs bring hope that this pattern can be broken, and that the risk of shingles can be considerably reduced, if not entirely eliminated. The first of these is a vaccine that has already proved highly effective in preventing chickenpox. The second is a stronger version of the same vaccine, which appears to cut in half the risk of shingles among adults who have already had chickenpox.

THE VARICELLA VACCINE

Regardless of whether or not vaccination against chickenpox will eventually prevent shingles, there are sound reasons for preventing chickenpox itself:

- Although chickenpox is considered mild compared with some other rash diseases, it nonetheless makes many children quite miserable, and costs their families much time and concern taking care of them.

- Not all individuals contract chickenpox during childhood. If they catch it as adolescents or adults, they are likely to be much sicker.
- Women who come down with chickenpox during pregnancy face a special risk. If they have the disease in early pregnancy, their babies may have serious birth defects. If they have it around the time of delivery, their babies may be severely infected with chickenpox, and may come down with shingles in childhood.
- Perhaps most important, a small but meaningful number of those who get chickenpox don't recover promptly or completely. The most common complication is secondary infection by bacteria, including a particularly nasty form of strep. Others include eye damage, pneumonia, and encephalitis, which are also potential complications of shingles (see chapter 5). Some individuals develop shingles itself in a relatively short time, rather than many years later.

The vaccine that prevents chickenpox is known formally as the **varicella vaccine**, named after the virus that causes chickenpox. It was first developed in the early 1970s by Japanese physician Michiaki Takahashi. The American pharmaceutical company Merck acquired rights to it in 1981, and after several years of extensive clinical tests, the Food and Drug Administration approved it for use in this country in 1995. It has been commercially available ever since, under the brand name Varivax.

As soon as the vaccine came into wide use, the number of children who caught chickenpox was dramatically reduced, and the percentage of those who became seriously ill was reduced even further. Originally, only a single shot was considered necessary, but there were still enough "breakthrough" cases—individuals who got chickenpox despite being vaccinated—that additional protection was sought. Pediatric experts now recommend a second, **booster shot**, administered anywhere from about three months to three years after the first.

Vaccination is now routine for children twelve months old or older. Many states require it before children can be admitted to public school. In the last couple of years, it has also been combined with others to form the so-called **MMRV** vaccine, active against measles, mumps, and rubella, as well as varicella.

The vaccine is a live but attenuated (weakened) form of the varicella virus. It has been biologically manipulated so that it remains alive, but is unable to reproduce well enough to cause disease. It retains enough of the features of the original virus for the vaccinated individual's immune system to recognize it and form antibodies to it. Thereafter, whenever the individual is exposed to the full-strength virus, the immune system will immediately react to it and keep it under control. In short, he or she will be immune to chickenpox.

The vaccine offers several benefits:

- A two-dose regimen completely prevents almost all chickenpox. It protects 98 percent of those vaccinated against any symptom-producing form of the disease.

- It also offers 100 percent protection against severe chickenpox. When vaccinated individuals do experience a **breakthrough infection**, it is much milder than usual. The fever is lower, the number of bumps is much smaller, and recovery is quicker.
- Those who do not catch chickenpox in the first place will not suffer its potentially serious complications, such as superimposed bacterial infections.

The vaccine also appears to provide good protection to non-immune individuals (such as family members) who are exposed to chickenpox, if it is administered within three days of the exposure.

The vaccine does not contain any mercury compounds or other preservatives. Neither does it contain any egg proteins, to which some individuals are allergic. Since it is a live vaccine, it must be kept frozen until it is ready for use. It is then diluted in a room-temperature solution, and must be injected within thirty minutes thereafter.

The vaccine itself is not known to cause any serious health problems, and its negative side effects are relatively few, minor, and temporary. The most common is inflammation at the injection site, with the typical symptoms of swelling, redness, and soreness. A low fever and a mild headache are also relatively common. Much rarer is an outbreak of rash, which may represent a low-level infection and may be contagious.

WHO SHOULD BE IMMUNIZED?

As we have said, the immunization of children and adolescents is now routine. It is also highly recommended for adults who have somehow managed to escape infection. It is considered especially advisable for certain groups, such as the following:

- Teachers, day-care workers, and others who are regularly in close contact with children.
- Health-care workers, who are in regular contact with the sick.
- Uninfected family members of individuals with chickenpox, as noted above.
- Individuals who live in close contact with one another, such as college students, prison inmates, and military personnel.
- Women of childbearing age, regardless of whether or not they have immediate plans to conceive. However, women who plan to become pregnant should be vaccinated at least one month beforehand, and certainly not once they are pregnant.
- Travelers to foreign countries.

There are exceptions. Some individuals are "contraindicated" (to use the medical jargon) for vaccination. That is, they are advised not to be vaccinated, or at least to delay vaccination until their medical conditions change. They include the following:

- Individuals suffering from an active, severe infectious illness, such as tuberculosis.
- Individuals who are allergic to components of the vaccine, such as gelatin and the antibiotic neomycin.
- Individuals who have within recent months received blood transfusions, or injections of blood products such as immune globulins.

- Pregnant women. The vaccine hasn't been proved harmless to developing fetuses. At the same time, there is no evidence that it has caused any damage when administered accidentally during pregnancy.
- Individuals with weakened immune systems from diseases such as lymphoma or AIDS, from corticosteroids, or from drugs used to prevent transplant rejection or to kill cancer cells.

This last category is no longer absolute. After all, individuals with weak immune systems are precisely those who are at greatest risk for catching chickenpox and are in greatest need of protection from it. The latest recommendations from the National Center for Immunization of the Centers for Disease Control and Prevention are that immunization of these individuals should not be routine, but should be reviewed by health professionals on a case-by-case basis. In many instances, the benefits of immunization may outweigh any potential risk.

WILL THE IMMUNITY LAST?

Infection with the varicella virus itself provides lifelong immunity to chickenpox. But will immunity provided by the weakened virus of the vaccine give equally long-lasting protection? Some health experts worry that if immunity wanes over time, those vaccinated in childhood might come down with the disease in adulthood, when it is likely to be more severe, and more likely to be followed by dangerous complications.

At present, there can be no absolute answer to this concern. As is true of all new vaccines, the full extent of protection offered by the varicella vaccine won't be known for decades. But with every passing year, there is additional evidence that immunization does provide enough protection to make it well worthwhile. In this country, the vaccine has been widely administered for more than ten years, and was clinically tested for several years before that. In Japan, the periods are even longer. There has been no statistical increase of chickenpox among adults since the vaccine was introduced. Moreover, even when breakthrough infections do occur, their severity is much reduced.

Tests for antibodies to the virus do exist, and theoretically it should be possible to identify vaccinated adults whose immunity has waned over time. However, the tests available for general use are not considered sensitive enough to be altogether reliable. Better tests may be developed in the future, or it may prove advisable to administer periodic booster shots during adulthood, as is done with some other vaccines.

BUT WILL IT STOP SHINGLES?

Public health authorities hope that varicella vaccination will become virtually universal, just as smallpox vaccination is. If it does, then chickenpox will eventually disappear, as smallpox has. And if chickenpox disappears, shingles should gradually disappear as well. If people don't get chickenpox, then the varicella zoster virus cannot become stored in their nerve roots. No virus, no shingles—at least in theory.

This prospect, cheery as it may be for future generations, probably offers little or no comfort to you who are reading this book. Almost certainly, you have already had chickenpox. If you haven't already had shingles, you run an increasing risk of getting it with every year you live. And even if you have already had shingles once, there is at least a slight chance that you will get it again. So, you might well ask, what can the varicella vaccine do for *me?*

The short-form answer is nothing. The vaccine used to prevent chickenpox will not prevent shingles among those who have already had chickenpox. But now there is available a much stronger form of the vaccine that shows meaningful promise in reducing the likelihood not only of shingles but also of post-herpetic neuralgia and other complications of shingles.

A month or so after he turned sixty, Nick Zarkoff had a thorough physical examination by his family doctor.

"You seem to be in pretty good shape," the doctor told him. "I want you to have some lab tests for confirmation, but I see no signs of any serious problem. Like most men your age, you'd do well to lose five or ten pounds, and you probably ought to be getting more regular exercise. But you don't smoke, and you drink moderately at most, so your outlook is good. Once we see what your cholesterol levels are, I might prescribe one of the statin drugs. But right now, all I would suggest is that you take one baby aspirin at least every other day to control blood clotting and reduce your risk of a heart attack or stroke."

"Is there anything else I ought to be doing for my health?" Nick asked.

"There is one thing that you might consider. Tell me, have you ever had chickenpox?"

"Well—sure. I had it when I was a kid—just about everybody I knew did. I got right over it, though."

"You got over it, but the virus that caused it never really went away. For many years, your immune system has kept it under control, but as you get older, your immune system gets weaker. And now that you're sixty, you are at greatly increased risk that the virus will become reactivated."

"I wouldn't get chickenpox again, would I?"

"No, you'll never get chickenpox again. But there's a good chance that you might come down with shingles."

"Shingles? Ouch! My brother-in-law had that a year ago. He was miserable for months."

"Shingles can be quite painful, and the pain may last. But now there's some hope that you can head it off, or at least make it less severe."

"Really? What's that?"

"There's a new vaccine out," said the doctor. "It isn't perfect, and I wish we knew more about how long it will keep working. But for someone your age, it appears to cut the risk of shingles by more than half. And even if you do get shingles, you're somewhat less likely to suffer from it as long or as much."

"Definitely worth considering," said Nick. "Can you tell me more?"

THE SHINGLES PREVENTION STUDY

At the same time that the varicella vaccine was demonstrating its effectiveness in preventing chickenpox, scientists at Merck were already exploring how the same weakened strain of the virus might be adapted for a vaccine to prevent shingles. They hypothesized that a much stronger dose might be able to raise the level of immunity high enough to keep the varicella zoster virus in the nerve roots from reactivating and proliferating.

Initial tests suggested that a vaccine fourteen times as strong as the one for chickenpox would achieve the best balance between safety and effectiveness. These preliminary tests were followed by a large clinical trial called the Shingles Prevention Study, which extended over several years and concluded in 2005.

The Shingles Prevention Study was carefully designed to produce clear and unambiguous results. It followed the criteria that have been established for trials of this kind.

- The number of volunteers tested was large—more than 38,000 in all. And the testing sites were located at hospitals and other medical centers all over the country.
- The subjects were carefully selected. For example, they had to be sixty years or older—the age group in which shingles is most prevalent. They had to be basically healthy. In particular, they couldn't have severe immune deficiencies as a result of disease or medical treatment. As a precaution, women of childbearing age were excluded.
- The subjects were then randomly assigned to two equal groups, each composed of about 19,000 individuals. The first group was injected with the experimental vaccine, and the second group received a **placebo**—a substance that looks exactly like the vaccine but doesn't contain its active ingredient.
- The study was **double blind**. Neither those giving nor those receiving the test injections knew which shots contained the vaccine and which contained only the placebo.

- The study continued for a significant period of time. Its subjects were monitored for an average of about three years—some for up to five years.

RESULTS OF THE STUDY

By 2005, the results of the study were plain. Those who received the vaccine were only about half as likely to have shingles as those who received the placebo. Moreover, those who were vaccinated and nonetheless came down with shingles tended to have somewhat milder symptoms and to recover a little sooner. More important, they were also at least somewhat less likely to develop post-herpetic neuralgia (PHN).

In May 2006, the Food and Drug Administration licensed the new vaccine, trade-named Zostavax, to help prevent shingles and its complications. The license applied only to the categories included in the Shingles Prevention Study—basically individuals aged sixty years or older whose immune systems were not unusually depressed. In October of the same year, the Advisory Committee on Immunization Practices (ACIP) of the Centers for Disease Control and Prevention recommended the vaccine for protection of the same population, increasing the likelihood that doctors would prescribe it and (perhaps just as important) that insurance companies would pay for it.

IT'S NOT PERFECT, BUT . . .

From a public-health point of view, the shingles vaccine offers great promise, especially if it becomes widely accepted and used. To reduce the number of people who suffer from shingles each year would offer significant public benefits in terms of saving money, regaining lost time, and generally improving quality of life. But for individuals and their doctors, the prospects are not so rosy. The vaccine does not offer complete protection from shingles; it just cuts down the risk. For many people, that may be good enough. But for those who are vaccinated and then come down with shingles anyway, the outcome is likely to be disappointing, to say the least.

Another potential drawback to the vaccine is reduced effectiveness among the very old. In the Shingles Reduction Study, the overall incidence of shingles was about 50 percent less in those who were vaccinated than in those who received a placebo. But that was for the total population of those tested. When the results were analyzed by age groups, dramatic differences showed up. Only among those aged 70 to 79 was the average reduction close to 50 percent. For those aged 60 to 69, the reduction was considerably greater—closer to two-thirds. But for those 80 or older, the reduction sank to a rather discouraging 18 percent. In short, those at highest risk for getting shingles benefited least from the vaccine.

So the choice of whether or not to receive the vaccine must be a personal one, which you and (hopefully) your doctor arrive at after carefully examining your particular situation. The vaccine is considered quite safe—the most common side effects are inflammation in the area of the injection and, sometimes, a relatively mild headache. On the other hand, the vaccine is fairly expensive, and at the time we are writing, insurance coverage for it is somewhat uncertain. The question that only you can answer is whether the potential benefits outweigh the expense.

We might as well admit it: Both of your authors took care to have ourselves immunized as soon as the vaccine became available. One of us had actually suffered from shingles and post-herpetic neuralgia in the past. Both of us ordered doses of the vaccine from pharmacists near our doctors' offices, and when they arrived, we made very specific appointments with our doctors and picked up the insulated packages a few minutes beforehand. Like the varicella vaccine, the shingles vaccine must be kept deeply frozen until it is to be used. So, within the thirty-minute window allowed, we delivered our doses to our doctors' offices, where they were immediately diluted, thawed, and injected.

We do not regret our decisions one bit. If either of us gets shingles at some point in the future, we won't be happy about it, but will take comfort in the thought that without the vaccine, we might suffer longer and more intensely. Sometimes half a loaf is indeed better than none.

WHO SHOULD—AND SHOULD NOT—BE IMMUNIZED?

The Shingles Prevention Study was designed to provide clear-cut results with minimum risk of adverse consequences for those tested. The current guidelines for immunization are based on that study. Several of them are similar to those for the chickenpox vaccine. Some of its restrictions seem obvious and well justified. Others appear to call for further study and possible re-evaluation.

Immunization is recommended for healthy individuals aged sixty or over. Exceptions include the following:

- Individuals suffering from an active, severe infectious illness, such as tuberculosis.
- Individuals who are allergic to components of the vaccine, such as gelatin and the antibiotic neomycin. (Incidentally, the vaccine contains no mercury compounds or other preservatives, nor any egg proteins.)
- Individuals who have within recent months received blood transfusions, or injections of blood products such as immune globulins.
- Individuals who are taking antiviral medications to treat other conditions caused by herpesviruses, such as herpes simplex 1 or 2. These medications might interfere with the shingles vaccine.
- Women of childbearing age. This guideline is far more stringent than that for the chickenpox vaccine, probably because the shingles vaccine is so much stronger. For older women, the restriction does not apply. But if immunization becomes available to women under sixty, the guideline may need to be re-examined.
- Individuals less than sixty years old. This guideline is based simply on the population of the Shingles Prevention Study, which was limited to those sixty and over. But about half of all shingles cases occur in people less than sixty, and the rate of incidence starts to rise sharply at about age fifty. Right now clinical trials are taking place to determine the effectiveness and safety of the vaccine among individuals fifty and older.
- Individuals with weakened immune systems from diseases such as lymphoma or AIDS, from corticosteroids, or from drugs used to prevent transplant rejection or to kill cancer cells. The same restriction

applies to the chickenpox vaccine, and, again, it is based upon caution. On the other hand, individuals with weak immune systems are at the greatest risk for getting shingles. Further tests may eventually reveal instances where the potential benefits of immunization outweigh the risks.

"How have you been feeling?" asked the neurologist who had been treating Estelle Freneaux's severe post-herpetic neuralgia for five months. "Any more attacks in the last couple of weeks?"

"Only a few twinges," Estelle replied. "Scary, but not really serious, and they don't last long. Knock on wood, but I think I'm about over this."

"You've been through a rough ordeal," said the doctor sympathetically. "PHN can be very hard to treat. Some patients just have to tough it out. You must be very relieved to have it over with."

"Very relieved. But I have a question for you. I'm almost afraid to ask it."

"What is it?"

"Am I through with this for good? Is there any chance I could get shingles again?"

"Not for at least three years, as far as we know. Having shingles boosts your immunity at least temporarily. But I have to be honest with you. The risk of recurrence is small, but it's there. About one in twenty patients eventually get it again."

"That's hard to face. Isn't there anything I can do about it?"

"There does exist a new vaccine for shingles. Nobody knows how well it would work on people like you, who have already had shingles. But even if you got it again, it would

probably be less serious. And you wouldn't be as likely to get PHN."

"Half a loaf, obviously," said Estelle, shrugging, "but better than none."

"I can't recommend it wholeheartedly," said the doctor. "We just don't know how long the immune protection will last."

"I don't care," said Estelle firmly. "I would do anything, anything, not to go through all this again."

"It would be pointless—maybe even counterproductive—for you to be vaccinated in less than three years from now," cautioned the doctor. "You have plenty of time to think it over."

QUESTIONS FOR THE FUTURE

As is true of any new medical treatment, there remain a number of unanswered questions that only time, clinical experience, and further testing can answer. The most important of these is the same one posed by the chickenpox vaccine: How long will the protection last? Already some experts suspect that chickenpox immunization will have to be supplemented by one or more booster shots in adulthood. Possibly the shingles vaccine will also need eventual reinforcement. But right now, it hasn't been in use long enough for anyone to know.

A related question is this: Will the vaccine help patients who have had shingles reduce the risk of getting it again? The vaccine has not been tested on this group, so the answer is still unknown.

A final question: Can the effectiveness of the shingles vaccine be improved, and the risk of shingles further diminished? The strength of the dose might be adjusted, for example, or the vaccination might be repeated after a short interval, as chickenpox vaccination now is. To find out whether any such changes would be effective or safe, extensive, controlled testing would be necessary.

In the long run, the best hope of preventing shingles probably lies with the chickenpox vaccine. If its use becomes almost universal, chickenpox could be wiped out, and shingles with it. Meanwhile, though, there are whole generations of us who caught chickenpox in childhood, and who run a greater risk of getting shingles with every year we live. For us, the shingles vaccine, with all its limitations, offers at least a chance of avoiding this painful and sometimes dangerous scourge.

QUESTIONS AND ANSWERS ABOUT SHINGLES

SHINGLES BASICS

If I come down with shingles, what kinds of symptoms can I expect?

There are two main symptoms. One is a patchy rash of small bumps that turn into blisters. The other is burning or stabbing pain in the area of the rash. It may begin before the rash appears, and may persist after the rash has healed.

Is it true that shingles only turns up on certain parts of the body?

Shingles can occur just about anywhere on the body. But it occurs most frequently on the trunk, especially near the waist (the name shingles comes from a word meaning "belt"). The second most common location is the face, especially the region of the forehead, eye, and nose.

When I had shingles, the rash was just a narrow band that ran from my breastbone around to my spine, on one side. Why did it appear in just that area?
Shingles is caused by inflammation of one or more sensory nerves (usually just one, or even a single branch of one) by the same virus that causes chickenpox. The sensory nerves are located in pairs along the spinal column, and each nerve of the pair serves a limited area on one side of the body. After a chickenpox infection, the virus survives, alive but inactive, in the root of the nerve, near the point of attachment to the spinal cord. When the virus reactivates, reproducing and spreading through the nerve, it produces pain and a skin rash in the specific area, or dermatome, served by the nerve. When you had shingles, it appeared in a single dermatome on your trunk.

I had chickenpox many years ago. I'm now in my sixties, and haven't had shingles, but I'm told that the older I get, the greater chance I have of getting it. Is that so?
As you get older, your immune system—your body's ability to recognize and defend itself from infection—becomes steadily weaker. Shingles apparently results when the immune system is no longer strong enough to prevent reactivation of the chickenpox virus in a nerve root. So the older you get, the greater your risk of shingles is.

My thirty-eight-year-old niece just came down with shingles. Isn't that unusual?
Shingles in younger people is uncommon, but it happens. Those most likely to get shingles are the immunosup-

pressed—people who lack the protection of a normal immune system. They include the following:

- Those who are taking drugs (chemotherapy) or receiving radiation for cancer. These treatments are intended to kill cancer cells, but they kill cells of the immune system as well.
- Those taking drugs intentionally designed to suppress the immune system, so as to prevent tissue rejection after an organ transplant.
- Those taking anti-inflammatory corticosteroids for diseases such as lupus or arthritis. These drugs weaken the immune system.
- Those who have blood diseases such as leukemia, lymphoma, or Hodgkin's disease, which naturally weaken the immune system.
- Those infected with HIV, the human immunovirus that attacks the immune system and causes AIDS.

In addition, for some individuals, younger or older, shingles is apparently triggered when the immune system is temporarily weakened by some acute disease, or by severe stress. And some come down with it for no apparent reason—"out of the blue."

If shingles is caused by the chickenpox virus, why would I get shingles rather than chickenpox later in life?

Apparently, once you have had chickenpox, your immunity to it remains strong enough to prevent another outbreak. But your immune system may not remain strong enough to prevent the reactivation of the virus that is hiding in a nerve root. That reactivated virus, confined within the nerve, is what causes shingles.

Does the shingles rash look like chickenpox?
Both the chickenpox and shingles rashes are made up of small bumps that turn into blisters. But the chickenpox rash is scattered over much of the body, while the shingles rash is usually limited to the area of a single dermatome. The shingles rash is also more concentrated, and the pain accompanying it is more severe than the itching of chickenpox.

How do I know if I have shingles?
About the only way you or your doctor can be sure you have shingles is to identify the rash when it appears. Symptoms that occur before that are often too vague or too easily mistaken for something else to make diagnosis certain.

However, you might consult your doctor if you experience a couple of telltale signs of the disease, other than a rash. The main one is tingling, itching, or pain in a limited area on one side of your body or face. The pain also tends to be distinctive: sharp, stabbing, or burning, and relieved somewhat by rest. And of course if you see any signs of a rash, you should get in touch with your doctor immediately.

Is a rash ever the first symptom of shingles?
Usually the rash appears only after other symptoms—even if the earlier symptoms are too vague to identify. The reactivation of the virus takes place in the nerve root, and it takes time—usually a couple of days—for the infec-

tion to move through the nerve fiber to the skin, where it produces the rash.

What is the usual course of the shingles rash?

The rash appears in successive, overlapping "crops." Each crop goes through four stages:

- *Papules*: small bumps on a reddish base
- *Vesicles*: blisters, filled with clear lymph fluid
- *Pustules*: enlarged blisters, filled with pus—lymph, white blood cells, and cell fragments
- *Scabs*: dry, crusted remains of pustules, after they have broken open

How long can I expect the shingles rash to last?
The rash usually lasts about a week to ten days from the time it first appears to the time that most of its scabs are crusted over. Complete healing of the skin may take a week or two longer.

Will the pain go away when the rash disappears?
Episodes of pain are likely to occur for another couple of weeks after the skin is healed. The normal duration of shingles is up to five weeks. If the pain persists or comes back after that, it is described as post-herpetic neuralgia.

If I get shingles, will it make me so sick that I have to go to bed?
Shingles varies widely in its severity. It may be so mild that it is hardly noticeable, or so severe that you are completely incapacitated. Even if you are able to continue

your ordinary activities, you may find that the pain is relieved by getting extra rest.

What are my chances of recovering completely from shingles?

Most people do recover completely, without any complications. Those seriously affected may suffer persistent pain—what's called post-herpetic neuralgia. Other possible complications are less common.

My wife had a terrible case of shingles last year. Is it at all likely that she'll get it again?

It is uncommon for anyone to have shingles more than once. The overall risk is about one in twenty, but most of those are people with extremely weak immune systems as a result of other disease, medical treatment, or advanced old age.

THE VARICELLA ZOSTER VIRUS

When I had shingles, my doctor said it was caused by the varicella zoster virus. What has that got to do with chickenpox?

The varicella zoster virus, or VZV for short, causes both chickenpox and shingles. Varicella is the medical name for chickenpox; zoster, the medical name for shingles.

When my husband had shingles, I discouraged my eighty-nine-year-old mother from visiting us, for fear she might catch it. Was I wrong to be concerned?

When you have shingles, you can't give shingles to anyone else. You can give chickenpox to someone who hasn't already had it, but the chances are that your mother had already had chickenpox.

My daughter, who works, has asked me to babysit my seven-year-old grandson while he's home with chickenpox. I know that I'm immune to chickenpox, since I had it myself years ago. But can I catch shingles from my grandson?

It is generally agreed that you can't catch shingles from someone with chickenpox. If you get shingles, the virus is your own, left over from the chickenpox you once had.

I get confused about germs. What's the difference between viruses and bacteria?

Bacteria are complete, living cells—like the cells in your body. Each cell has a nucleus, containing chainlike molecules of DNA that carry the genetic code for reproduction. Bacteria can reproduce and multiply on their own.

The particles of a virus are much smaller and simpler. Each virus particle has two basic parts. One is a single length of either DNA or a similar molecule called RNA. The other is a coating of protein. Viruses cannot reproduce on their own. Virus particles must invade living cells and take over their reproductive machinery, so they can produce more virus. The new virus particles can then migrate from the host cells to invade other cells, spreading the infection.

In practical terms, the main difference between bacterial and viral infections is the way they are treated. Bacterial infections are treated with antibiotics, which kill bacterial cells. Antibiotics are ineffective against viruses. Viral diseases are treated with antiviral drugs, which hinder reproduction of the virus. Also, many viral diseases can be prevented with vaccines, which strengthen the immune system against specific viruses.

My doctor tells me that the chickenpox virus is related to the viruses that cause cold sores and genital herpes. How is that?

VZV is one of the herpesviruses. Other viruses in this group cause cold sores, genital herpes, and mononucleosis. They have several traits in common. They only reproduce in human cells. They are extremely contagious. They never completely die out in their human hosts, although their effects may be controlled by the hosts' immune systems.

How does the immune system work?

Your immune system is made up of different kinds of white blood cells, plus certain chemicals they produce. It has two basic mechanisms. It attacks any substances in your body that have been identified as foreign, and either destroys them or makes them inactive. It also learns to recognize many specific foreign substances the first time they enter your body, so they can be attacked even faster and more effectively if they ever appear again.

How is it that I became immune to chickenpox, but only after I had the disease?

When you were first infected by the chickenpox virus (probably when you were a child) your immune system didn't recognize it, and was relatively slow in mounting a counterattack against it. So you had to suffer chickenpox for a few days, until your immune system got control of it.

In the process, your immune system did learn to recognize the virus. Whenever you were exposed to it again,
your immune system attacked it immediately and effectively, so you've never again had chickenpox.

Why do most people catch chickenpox in childhood, rather than later on?

The virus is extremely contagious. Its particles are easily
passed on, mainly in small droplets of moisture that are
breathed out by the infected person, starting even before
any obvious symptoms appear.

Up until about a decade ago, when one child in a household, a day-care center, or a classroom got chickenpox, it was
very likely that others would catch it as well. As a result,
most children got chickenpox before they were adolescents.

Since the mid-1990s, however, a vaccine has sharply reduced the number of cases of chickenpox. It shows promise
of eventually eliminating almost all incidence of the disease.

When I had shingles, I was so sick I had to go to the hospital for a few days. One of the nurses had never had chickenpox and had never received the vaccine against it. She wasn't permitted to care for me. Why was that?

For children, chickenpox is usually (though not always) a
mild disease. But individuals who don't catch it until they
are adolescents or adults are likely to suffer more severe
attacks, and are at greater risk for dangerous complications. When you had shingles, your blisters contained particles of virus, and you could have given chickenpox to the
nurse who had never had it and who wasn't yet immunized against it. So she was told to avoid contact with you.

Is it true that even though I am immune to chicken-pox, there's still some of the virus in my body?

The varicella zoster virus, like other herpesviruses, never completely dies out in the body. Your immune system prevents it from causing chickenpox ever again. But the virus "hides out" in the roots of sensory nerves, and may eventually cause shingles.

For years I've suffered from recurrent cold sores on my upper lip. I understand that they are caused by a virus that is related to the virus for chickenpox and shingles. Why is it that cold sores keep coming back, but chickenpox and shingles occur just once each?

Herpes simplex type 1, which causes cold sores, is less well controlled by the immune system than is the varicella zoster virus, following a first infection. So cold sores keep coming back periodically, although later attacks tend to be less serious than the first one.

The immune system usually provides permanent immunity to chickenpox. But it may not remain able to prevent the virus in the nerve roots from reactivating and causing shingles. But shingles itself seems to restore the ability of the immune system to recognize and attack the virus, so that a repeat attack is uncommon.

SHINGLES TREATMENT

When my father had shingles, friends recommended all sorts of folk remedies for it. What are now considered the most effective forms of treatment?

Only in recent times has much been known about shingles and its causes. Before that, a lot of different remedies were tried, and most of them didn't work. Now there are two main forms of treatment:

- *Antiviral drugs*, which directly attack the virus that causes the disease.
- *Palliative remedies*, which relieve the symptoms of the disease even if they don't affect its course. These include painkillers of various kinds, and techniques to reduce psychological stress.

I've heard that if I get shingles, I should seek treatment right away. Aside from making me more comfortable, why is that so important?

The first line of defense against shingles is antiviral drugs, and they must be taken early in the course of the disease to be fully effective.

How do antiviral drugs work? Do they kill the virus?

Antiviral drugs don't kill the virus, the way that antibiotics kill bacteria. Instead, they stop it from reproducing, so it does less harm. They change the form of the DNA molecule of the virus, so that it can't completely copy itself. But the existing virus survives, until the immune system eventually gets control of it. So the earlier treatment with antiviral drugs starts, the less the virus accumulates in the nerve. The disease won't last as long, and its symptoms are likely to be less severe.

My neighbor said that when she had shingles, she didn't even call her doctor because the rash hardly bothered her. Was that wise?

She was taking a chance that the attack would soon resolve itself without treatment. Antiviral drugs, which must be prescribed by a doctor, are recommended for anyone who has shingles, even if the attack is mild.

What are the antiviral drugs most widely used for shingles?

There are three antiviral drugs commonly used for shingles. The oldest is acyclovir, which is taken both by injection (intravenously) and by mouth. The brand name of the pill form is Zovirax. The other two, taken only by mouth, are famciclovir (brand name Famvir) and valacyclovir (Valtrex).

If I take an antiviral drug, do I have to worry about serious side effects?

Antiviral drugs act selectively upon the virus, and have little or no effect on normal cells. Their side effects are usually no more than mildly annoying. The most common are headache and digestive-tract irritations—nausea, and either constipation or diarrhea. Less common is irritation of the kidneys. You should of course report any side effects to your doctor, but they are seldom troublesome enough to make you stop taking the drug.

What drugs can I take to relieve the pain of shingles?

There are essentially four types of painkillers used to make shingles pain more tolerable:

- nonsteroidal anti-inflammatory drugs (NSAIDs), such as aspirin and ibuprofen;
- acetaminophen, of which the best-known form is Tylenol;
- corticosteroids, sometimes called simply steroids; and
- narcotics, also known as opioids.

I get confused by all the different painkillers sold over the counter. For instance, what's the difference between aspirin and ibuprofen?

Aspirin and ibuprofen differ slightly in their chemical composition, but they work in similar ways. They are the only over-the-counter drugs in a group called non-steroidal anti-inflammatory drugs, or NSAIDs. That is, they relieve inflammation, but they aren't steroids. They also seem to affect the perception of pain in the central nervous system.

Aspirin and ibuprofen seem to upset my stomach, and my doctor recommends acetaminophen instead. Does it work differently from aspirin and ibuprofen?

Among the possible side effects of NSAIDs is irritation of the stomach lining, sometimes to the extent of causing ulcers and bleeding. Acetaminophen affects only the central perception of pain. It doesn't relieve inflammation, but it doesn't irritate the stomach, either. Its principal danger, when taken in large doses over a period of time, is damage to the liver or kidneys.

The best-known brand of acetaminophen is Tylenol. Some over-the-counter formulations, such as Excedrin, contain both acetaminophen and aspirin.

When I had shingles, my doctor gave me prescriptions for both an antiviral drug and prednisone—a steroid. He warned me not to take the steroid without taking the antiviral. Why was that?

Steroids, more accurately called corticosteroids, are effective in relieving the inflammation that produces the pain and itching of shingles. But these drugs have some undesirable side effects, including a tendency to suppress your immune system. Even while they are relieving the symptoms of shingles, they may be reinforcing one of its underlying causes. Most medical experts now feel that the benefits outweigh the risks, but they agree that corticosteroids should always be taken with antivirals, which directly attack the main cause of the disease.

Are the steroids used to fight inflammation the same as those that athletes take to bulk themselves up?
The term steroid is confusing. As popularly used, it refers both to the corticosteroid drugs used to relieve inflammation, and to the anabolic steroids used (and abused) to improve athletic performance. The two have nothing in common.

My shingles pain was so bad my doctor recommended a narcotic, but I was scared of becoming addicted, so I wouldn't take it. Was I right?
Narcotics are among the most effective painkillers known. They are also called opioids, because they are either derived from opium or chemically similar to it. Taken in large amounts in order to get high, they can lead to addiction. But taken in moderate amounts, under medical supervision, to relieve physical pain, they seldom if ever cause such problems.

Also, opioids vary a lot in their potency. Those prescribed for shingles are usually mild varieties, such as codeine or propoxyphene (brand name Darvon).

I've heard that shingles is sometimes more itchy than painful. What sort of treatment is given for that?
Topical anti-itch medications (known formally as antiprurients) are used to relieve the intense itching that

shingles sometimes causes. One that you are doubtlessly familiar with is calamine lotion. Others are ointments containing topical anesthetics such as lidocaine or prilocaine.

Unfortunately, widely used salves and ointments based on antihistamines and corticosteroids are not as effective against the itching of shingles.

When my aunt had shingles, her doctor suggested that she crush some aspirin tablets into powder, mix it with rubbing alcohol, and dab it on the rash. It really seemed to help. Is this a common remedy?
Combining crushed aspirin and evaporating fluid is a home remedy of long standing. It does appear to give at least temporary relief to some patients.

Would the kind of ointment used for insect bites and burns give any relief from shingles?
A common type of ointment for painful skin conditions has as its active ingredient a topical anesthetic, such as lidocaine, prilocaine, or pramoxine. It doesn't just suppress pain; it makes the skin numb, and can provide very welcome temporary relief.

When my neighbor had shingles, she started doing some exercises to reduce psychological stress. What has shingles got to do with stress?
Pain of many kinds can be triggered or intensified by psychological stress. Conversely, the reduction of stress can actually relieve the perception of pain. Stress-reducing techniques can reinforce the effects of drugs and other medical agents in relieving shingles pain.

I have long used a technique called progressive relaxation to help me get to sleep. I concentrate on specific muscle groups in my body, from my feet to my forehead, and imagine them as comfortable and relaxed. I've heard that the same technique can be used to help cope with pain. Is that so?
One of the best ways to control psychological stress is by achieving physical relaxation. Some psychologists believe that it is impossible to be both physically relaxed and psychologically tense at the same time. To be effective, relaxation exercises have to be practiced regularly until they become habitual.

A friend at work says that meditation helped him a lot when he got shingles. How does it work?
Meditation is an ancient technique of mental distraction. Its traditional function is to separate the mind from the limits of ordinary reality and to achieve inner peace. But it can also reduce stress and pain, by distracting your attention away from them. It is performed by sitting or lying in a relaxed position, repeating a single word over and over, and allowing your mind to become as empty and passive as possible.

I've heard that mental techniques called directed imagery and sensory substitution are used to relieve shingles pain. What are they?
Both are techniques that use the power of imagination to divert attention from pain or to reshape the perception of it. Guided imagery involves forming a mental image of a pleasant, tranquil scene and then immersing yourself entirely in it until you are free of stress and the conscious-

ness of pain. Sensory substitution is imagining that a painful sensation has been replaced with some other, nonpainful one, such as coolness or mild prickling. Like other methods of stress control, these techniques can only be mastered through concentration and repeated practice.

When the pain of shingles on my chest kept me from sleeping, my doctor recommended wrapping the area with an elastic sports bandage. It really did help—but how did it work?

What your doctor recommended was a simple application of a natural process of pain relief called counterirritation. The mildly irritating sensations produced by the pressure of the elastic bandage are transmitted to the central nervous system, where they trigger reactions that diminish the perception of pain. Another form of counterirritation that sometimes helps with shingles is a liniment such as oil of wintergreen, which initially makes the skin feel warm.

When my cousin had shingles, she was given something called a TENS unit to help relieve her pain. It used electricity in some way. What was it?

Transcutaneous electrical nerve stimulation, or TENS for short, is most often used to treat joint and muscle pain, but it is also occasionally used to relieve shingles. A portable machine produces mild pulses of electrical current which pass through electrodes to the skin, provoking a tingling sensation. Just how it works and how effective it is are subjects of dispute, but some people get at least some relief from it.

POST-HERPETIC NEURALGIA

After suffering miserably from shingles, I thought the pain would go away not long after the rash disappeared. Instead, I'm still in lots of pain. What's the matter?
Unfortunately, you have what is called post-herpetic neuralgia—PHN for short. It is the most common complication of shingles, and it is defined as significant pain that persists or returns after the shingles rash heals and disappears.

I'm just getting over shingles. A friend of mine who had it six months ago is still in serious pain. What are my chances of going through the same thing?
Nobody can predict exactly who will get PHN after shingles. But certain factors seem to raise the risk:

- *Severe shingles.* If you have a severe attack of shingles, and especially if you suffered significant pain before the rash appeared, you are more likely to get PHN.
- *Increasing age.* The older you are when you have shingles, the more likely you are to suffer PHN afterward.
- *Extreme immunosuppression.* Individuals with greatly weakened immune systems, from disease or medical treatment, are more likely to suffer PHN after shingles.

If I do get PHN after I recover from shingles, how long will it last and how much will I suffer?
PHN, like shingles itself, varies enormously. For some, it is no more than a minor annoyance; for others, it is a dis-

abling misery. Most people get over it within a few weeks or months; for an unfortunate minority, the pain may continue indefinitely.

I was told that once the shingles rash heals, the virus is no longer active. So why does the pain persist?
Apparently, the acute attack of the virus causes lasting damage to nerve cells, and this damage in turn causes pain sensations even after the virus has become inactive.

Is it possible to get PIIN without having shingles first?
PHN is a direct consequence of shingles. It doesn't occur on its own.

Mostly, the pain I have now is the same as when I had shingles. But there's also something new. The lightest touch—just wearing a shirt—can set off awful stabs of pain. What's going on?
The mysterious and very distressing symptom called allodynia is somewhat more typical of PHN than of shingles. Allodynia is pain triggered by some sensation that is not in itself painful—such as a light, moving touch across the skin. Apparently the harmless sensation, transmitted through nerves that don't normally sense pain, somehow triggers the nerves that do transmit pain sensations.

This continuing pain really wears me down. I get very little sleep. I've lost my appetite. I don't want to go anywhere or see anybody. Is this common?
Even more than shingles, PHN can be physically and emotionally debilitating. Insomnia, loss of appetite, depression, and social withdrawal are indeed common. Fortunately, there are many forms of treatment, both physical

and psychological, now available to help you manage these consequences of pain.

I took an antiviral drug when I first came down with shingles, but my doctor says it won't work against PHN. Is that so?

Antiviral drugs are only helpful at an early stage of shingles, when they prevent the virus from reproducing further. PHN occurs after the virus has become inactive, so antivirals have no effect on it.

My doctor tells me that the aspirin and codeine I took when I had shingles probably won't be as helpful now that I have PHN. Is she right?

The painkillers commonly used to relieve the pain of shingles—aspirin and other nonsteroidal anti-inflammatory drugs (NSAIDs), acetaminophen (Tylenol), and mild narcotics such as codeine—are not strong enough to relieve the pain of PHN.

I've heard that the pain that follows shingles is now often treated with antidepressant drugs. Is that because the pain causes depression?

Just as antiviral drugs have become leading tools in relieving shingles, so antidepressants have become leading tools in relieving PHN. Specific antidepressants known as tricyclics are used to treat PHN, but they are given in smaller doses than those used to treat depression. They apparently work by hindering the transmission of pain impulses to the brain.

If I take an antidepressant for PHN, what side effects do I have to worry about?

The side effects of antidepressants, especially when taken in small doses, are usually no more than mildly annoying. Probably the most common is dryness of the mouth, and the next most common is constipation. Other possible nuisances include "cold" sweating, drowsiness, susceptibility to fainting, heart palpitations, and weight gain from increased appetite.

Is it true that drugs used for epileptic seizures are also used for PHN?
Anticonvulsant drugs are used to control the abnormal activity in brain cells that produces the convulsions of epilepsy. They can also be useful in controlling spasms of stabbing pain in PHN, especially those triggered by non-painful sensations (allodynia).

What was the special ointment my aunt was given for the pain she had after shingles? It burned like the dickens when she first put it on, but after a while she got used to it, and it did give her some relief.
A topical ointment sometimes used for PHN is based on capsaicin—the active ingredient in hot peppers. Capsaicin is thought to lower the level of a chemical that enhances the transmission of pain impulses to the central nervous system. When first applied to the skin, it produces a burning, stinging sensation, which is followed by at least some reduction in sensitivity to pain.

A friend of mine says he found biofeedback helpful in controlling the pain he had following shingles. How does it work?
Relaxation helps to relieve pain by reducing stress. Biofeedback might be described as mechanically assisted

relaxation. It is a machine that registers physical signs of stress and makes them audible or visible. The higher the level of stress, the stronger the output. Apparently, when you become more aware of your level of stress, you are better able to control it and achieve relaxation.

Hypnosis is sometimes used to treat painful conditions like chronic headaches. Might it help relieve PHN?

Hypnosis is occasionally used in efforts to relieve stubborn PHN. In a hypnotic trance you become strongly susceptible to suggestion, which can greatly alter your perception—including the perception of pain. Hypnotic suggestion can make a part of your body numb, or make a painful sensation feel like some other, nonpainful one (sensory substitution). The effects may persist after you emerge from the trance—a phenomenon called posthypnotic suggestion. The big drawback to hypnosis is that many people are not capable of being hypnotized.

A friend at work has been on disability for months for the pain he's suffered ever since he had shingles. Recently he's been advised to get psychotherapy. Would that really help with his pain?

Such forms of psychotherapy as cognitive therapy and behavioral therapy are sometimes helpful in relieving persistent PHN. Psychotherapy may not directly relieve pain, but may help keep it from intensifying in the downward spiral of what's called a "pain cycle," in which pain leads to stress, which leads to more pain, and so forth. Just as important, therapy can help patients cope better with pain, so that it doesn't become completely disabling.

I've heard that something called a nerve block can stop pain sensation completely. Would that be helpful with PHN?

Nerve blocks completely stop the transmission of impulses. They are sometimes used to treat PHN, usually as a last resort, when the pain is severe and long lasting, and other approaches have failed. They have many potentially serious side effects, and even the most radical of them—completely severing the nerves—offers only temporary relief.

My sister has a very capable doctor, but so far the things he's done for the pain she's had since getting shingles aren't much help. Now he's suggesting she try the pain clinic at the university medical center. What's the advantage of that?

Pain clinics, often associated with a teaching hospital or university medical school, use a team of experts that might include a neurologist, an anesthesiologist, a physical therapist, and a psychologist, among others. The team prepares a systematic treatment plan, often involving several different forms of treatment at once. The goals are not only to reduce pain and speed recovery, but also to restore normal function. The combination of physical and psychological approaches can help patients cope with their condition and carry on with their lives, even if they haven't completely recovered.

I think I'm beginning to feel a little better. What will my recovery from PHN be like?

Attacks of pain will alternate with periods of relief, and the attacks will gradually become shorter and less intense, while the pain-free periods become longer. The process may extend for months, but once the pattern becomes established, you can at least be reassured that eventual recovery is on the way.

OTHER COMPLICATIONS OF SHINGLES

I thought shingles appeared mainly around the middle of the body, but my father-in-law has it on his upper face. Is that common?
Shingles does occur most often in various parts of the trunk, especially the dermatomes close to the waist. But the dermatome of the upper face, from the forehead to the end of the nose, is the most common single site of the disease, accounting for about 15 percent of all cases.

I've just been to my doctor for a bad headache on one side of my head. I thought it might be a migraine. He got all concerned when he spotted a little patch of rash near the tip of my nose, and wants me to see an ophthalmologist right away. What's the problem?
A patch of rash near the tip of the nose, called Hutchinson's sign, is considered early evidence of shingles originating in the upper, or ophthalmic, branch of the trigeminal nerve in the face. This form of shingles is called herpes zoster ophthalmicus, or HZO for short. Its particular danger is that the viral infection may spread to the eye, so it is advisable to have an ophthalmologist as part of the treatment team.

When my brother first showed signs of shingles near his eye, his doctor started treatment that very day. What kind of harm can shingles do to the eye?

HZO is considered especially dangerous because the eye is a delicate organ and quite susceptible to damage. The viral infection can affect just about any part of the eye, and the damage it causes may be irreversible. It may even eventually cause the diminishment or complete loss of vision in the affected eye. That's why prompt treatment of HZO is so crucial.

Herpes near the eye is sure unsightly. My sister-in-law's eyelids—especially the upper one—are swollen almost shut, as if she's been slugged in the eye. She refuses to go out—can't bear to be seen. Will all this go away?

Inflammation of the eyelids is a very common consequence of HZO, and it usually subsides when the acute attack ends. But severe inflammation may permanently damage the lids so that some of the lashes are lost, or the lids don't close properly.

Shingles has given my uncle a bad case of pinkeye. It hurts him a lot. Will it do any permanent harm?

The virus often inflames the conjunctiva, a transparent membrane over the white of the eye, or the sclera, the white of the eye, or the other outer layers of the eyeball. The inflammation may be very painful, but usually subsides without causing permanent damage.

When an ophthalmologist examined my eye after I came down with shingles, she said that she was looking for signs of keratitis. What's that?

Keratitis is an inflammation of the cornea, a kind of transparent window in the front part of the eye. Keratitis is a common complication of HZO, and it can lead either directly or by secondary bacterial infection to permanent ulceration or scarring that harms vision.

I've heard that shingles of the eye can cause glaucoma, and I know that glaucoma can cause blindness. Is this a serious risk?
Glaucoma is caused by abnormally high pressure of the fluids in the eyeball. The pressure can gradually damage the optic nerve, leading to "tunnel" vision, or, in extreme cases, blindness. The inflammation of HZO can sometimes lead to an increase in this intraocular pressure, and it's fairly easy to check. So that's one of the things an ophthalmologist looks for when you get HZO.

Besides cornea damage and the risk of glaucoma, are there any other big threats to the eye from HZO?
The main dangers include cataracts in the lens and inflammation of the eyeball lining, the retina, or the optic nerve. Almost any part of the eye can be affected, which is why careful monitoring and prompt treatment are so important.

What's the main treatment for HZO?
Like other forms of shingles, HZO should be treated with antiviral drugs as early as possible. It's the best way to reduce the risk of eye involvement.

Is HZO treated any differently from other kinds of shingles?
The main difference in treatment is a greater willingness to use corticosteroids to fight inflammation. The side effects of steroids make some doctors reluctant to prescribe

them, but the potential risks of eye inflammation are so high that many feel that the benefits outweigh the risks.

If my ophthalmologist finds signs of increased pressure in my eye, can anything be done to head off glaucoma?
Glaucoma can usually be controlled with drugs, many applied as eyedrops. Some decrease the production of fluid in the eye; others help the drainage of excess fluid. In extreme cases, surgery may be needed to prevent fluid buildup.

If parts of the eye become severely damaged by HZO, can anything be done to repair them?
Severe damage is uncommon, but it can often be repaired by surgery. A badly scarred cornea, for example, can be replaced with a human transplant, and a lens with a serious cataract can be replaced with an artificial substitute.

My next-door neighbor had a very strange kind of shingles. It seemed to be centered in his ear, and it temporarily damaged his hearing. But the really strange thing was that the muscles in the side of his face were paralyzed. What did he have?
Shingles in the so-called facial nerve often affects other nearby nerves, causing a group of symptoms called Ramsay Hunt syndrome. The symptoms include earache, rash in or around the ear, loss of taste in part of the tongue, loss of hearing, dizziness, and paralysis of facial muscles. Most of them pass off with the acute infection, but the facial paralysis and hearing loss may linger for some time.

I know that as a rule the chickenpox rash appears over much of the body, while shingles turns up in just one area. Does shingles ever "escape" to other parts of the body?

Shingles is usually confined to a single dermatome. Only rarely does it spread, or disseminate, elsewhere. Disseminated shingles occurs almost entirely in individuals who are severely immunosuppressed. It can be very dangerous, for unlike ordinary shingles, it can affect internal organs, causing pneumonia in the lungs, or inflammation of the brain and its membranes (encephalitis).

VACCINES TO PREVENT CHICKENPOX AND SHINGLES

Is there really an effective way of preventing chickenpox?

Since 1995, the varicella vaccine (brand name Varivax) has greatly reduced chickenpox in this country. Its use is now routine, and many states require vaccination before a child is admitted to school. Current recommendations call for two shots; the first given at twelve months, the second up to three years or so later. These prevent almost all chickenpox and stop virtually all severe attacks.

Chickenpox is a fairly mild disease. Is it really worthwhile to be immunized against it?

There are several good reasons for preventing chickenpox. For example:

- Chickenpox varies a lot in severity. Even small children may be made quite miserable by it. And those who don't catch it until they are adolescents or adults are likely to suffer severe attacks.

- Women who come down with chickenpox during pregnancy face special risks. If they have the disease in early pregnancy, their babies may have serious birth defects. If they have it around the time of delivery, their babies may be severely infected with chickenpox and may come down with shingles in childhood.
- Some people who get chickenpox don't recover promptly or completely. In particular, they may suffer a secondary infection by bacteria.
- Only those who have had chickenpox get shingles later in life. Preventing chickenpox offers the best hope of preventing shingles.

What exactly is a vaccine? How does it protect you from a virus?

A vaccine is a chemical substance that is either derived from a particular virus or resembles it closely. When it is injected into your body, the look-alike won't cause disease, but it will "fool" your immune system into developing antibodies to the real virus. Thereafter, if you are infected by the virus, the antibodies will attach themselves to it and mark it for quick destruction by other parts of your immune system. In short, you are now immune to that virus.

How is the varicella vaccine produced?

The varicella vaccine is an attenuated (weakened) form of the virus. That is, the virus has been manipulated so it can't multiply and cause disease. But it is enough like the full-strength virus that the immune system will develop antibodies to the virus.

Is the vaccine safe? Does it have any significant side effects?

The vaccine is not known to cause any serious health problems, and its possible side effects are relatively mild. The most common is inflammation (redness, swelling, and tenderness) at the site of the shot. Less common are a low fever and a mild headache. Rarer still is an outbreak of rash, which may represent a low-level chickenpox infection.

Is there anybody who shouldn't get the varicella vaccine?

There are some individuals for whom the vaccine isn't recommended. They include:

- Those who have an active infectious disease such as tuberculosis.
- Those who are allergic to vaccine components, such as gelatin and the antibiotic neomycin.
- Those who have recently received blood transfusions or injections of immune globulins.
- Pregnant women. The vaccine hasn't been proved harmless to a developing fetus.
- Those who have weakened immune systems.

Why isn't the vaccine recommended for people who have weak immune systems? Aren't they just the ones who need it most?

The reason is caution. Medical authorities worry that if an individual has a very weak immune system, the vaccine may not produce immunity, but may instead make the person even more susceptible to infection.

However, the National Center for Immunization of the Centers for Disease Control and Prevention now recommends that immunizing such individuals should be reviewed on a case-by-case basis. For some, the benefits of immunization may outweigh the risks.

How can we be sure that people who get the varicella vaccine not only won't get chickenpox, but won't come down with shingles later on?
It will take decades to prove for sure that the vaccine will provide long-term protection against chickenpox. But every passing year gives additional evidence that the protection is indeed lasting. And preventing chickenpox appears to be the best way to prevent shingles later on.

I've already had chickenpox. What can the varicella vaccine do for *me*?
Nothing, unfortunately. But a new vaccine, recently approved, shows promise in preventing shingles or at least making its effects less severe.

How does the varicella vaccine for chickenpox differ from the zoster vaccine for shingles?
Both are based on the same attenuated (weakened) form of the live virus. But the zoster vaccine (brand name Vostavax) is fourteen times stronger than the varicella vaccine.

How effective is the zoster vaccine, compared to the varicella vaccine?
It is not as effective. Two doses of the varicella vaccine prevent almost all chickenpox. In the large clinical trial

that preceded the approval of the zoster vaccine, the risk of shingles was reduced about 50 percent overall. But the reduction varied a lot by age. Only for those 70 to 79 years old was the reduction close to 50 percent. For those 60 to 69, the reduction was higher—almost two-thirds. But for those 80 or more, the percentage dropped to just 18 percent. In short, the older you are when you receive the vaccine, the less effective it is likely to be.

Does the zoster vaccine make shingles less severe? Does it prevent post-herpetic neuralgia?

The clinical trial showed that those who did get shingles tended to have less severe symptoms and to recover faster. And there was a significant reduction in the risk of getting post-herpetic neuralgia afterward.

Is the zoster vaccine safe? Does it have any significant side effects?

It appears to be safe for those on whom it has been fully tested—basically healthy individuals, aged sixty or older. Its side effects are mild. Like the varicella vaccine, it may produce some local inflammation at the site of the shot. And you might experience a slight, temporary headache.

Who should—and should not—receive the zoster vaccine?

At present, immunization is recommended for healthy individuals aged sixty or over. Exceptions include the following:

- Individuals who have an active, severe infectious disease, such as tuberculosis.
- Individuals who are allergic to vaccine components such as gelatin and neomycin.

- Individuals who have recently received blood transfusions or injections of blood products such as immune globulins.
- Individuals who are taking antiviral drugs for other herpesvirus conditions.
- Women of childbearing age.
- Individuals younger than sixty years old.
- Individuals with weakened immune systems.

Why should women of childbearing age, individuals younger than sixty, and individuals with weakened immune systems be stopped from getting the vaccine?
Caution, mainly. These categories were excluded from the big clinical trial on which FDA approval was based. Health authorities feel that further controlled tests are needed before the current recommendations are further relaxed.

Will the zoster vaccine provide lasting immunity? Will it provide extra protection to those who have already had shingles?
The answers to these questions are not known. The first can be answered only after enough years pass to determine whether "breakthrough" infections occur at a higher rate than might have been expected among those who have been immunized. The second can probably be answered through further controlled testing.

GLOSSARY

acetaminophen (*ah-seet-ah-MIN-oh-fen*). Brand name
Tylenol, and many generics. Over-the-counter analgesic
(pain reliever) that alters the perception of pain in the
central nervous system. Acetominophen has fewer potentially harmful side effects than aspirin and other
nonsteroidal anti-inflammatory drugs (NSAIDs).

acetylsalicylic (*ah-SEE-til-sal-ih-sil-ik*) **acid**. Medical
name for aspirin. *See also* nonsteroidal anti-inflammatory drugs.

acoustic nerve. Cranial nerve that registers the sensations of hearing and balance. Shingles in this and other
nearby cranial nerves can cause a condition known as
Ramsay Hunt syndrome. *See also* cranial nerves, Ramsay Hunt syndrome.

acute retinal necrosis (*RET-ih-nahl nek-ROH-sis*). Inflammation of the retina of the eye caused by herpes
zoster ophthalmicus. It may lead to vision-threatening
detachment (separation) of the retina from the lining

of the eyeball. *See also* herpes zoster ophthalmicus, retina.

acyclovir (*ay-SYE-kloh-veer*). Brand name Zovirax (*ZOH-vir-aks*). Antiviral drug, taken orally (by mouth) or intravenously (by injection). *See also* antiviral drugs.

Advil. Brand name for ibuprofen.

AIDS. Abbreviation for acquired immune deficiency syndrome. *See also* HIV.

allodynia (*al-oh-DIN-ee-ah*). Neurogenic pain, triggered by some sensation that is not in itself painful, such as a light, moving touch across the skin. Allodynia is more typical of post-herpetic neuralgia (PHN) than of shingles. *See also* neurogenic pain.

analgesic. A drug that relieves pain. *See also* acetaminophen, nonsteroidal anti-inflammatory drugs, narcotics.

anesthetic. A drug that inhibits sensation. Topical anesthetics, applied to the skin surface, and local anesthetics, injected into specific parts of the body, cause numbness in the areas where they are applied. General anesthetics cause loss of consciousness as well as sensation.

antibiotics. Drugs used to treat or prevent infection by bacteria. Antibiotics are ineffective against shingles, which is caused by a virus. They are sometimes given to shingles patients to prevent secondary bacterial infection.

antibodies. Protein molecules produced by certain white blood cells of the immune system. Antibodies attach themselves to foreign invaders, marking them for destruction by other immune cells. Also known as immune globulins and immunoglobulins. *See also* varicella zoster immune globulin.

anticonvulsants. Drugs mainly used to treat epileptic seizures, but also used to relieve post-herpetic neuralgia (PHN). Anticonvulsants are often prescribed for allodynia, which is thought to be caused by the uncontrolled, abnormal firing of pain-sensing neurons. *See also* allodynia, gabapentin, pregabalin.

antidepressants. Drugs mainly used to relieve psychological depression, but administered in smaller doses to relieve post-herpetic neuralgia (PHN). They apparently enhance the activity of chemical neurotransmitters in spinal nerves that hinder the transmission of pain impulses to the brain. *See also* desipramine, neurotransmitters, nortriptyline, tricyclic antidepressants.

antiprurients. Anti-itch medications.

antiviral drugs. Drugs used to control virus attacks. They do not kill the virus, but stop it from reproducing. Antivirals act selectively upon the virus, and have little or no effect on normal cells. *See also* acyclovir, famciclovir, valacyclovir.

ASA. Abbreviation for acetylsalicylic acid.

attenuated virus. Biologically manipulated virus that cannot reproduce well enough to cause disease, and so can be used as a vaccine. *See also* vaccine.

axon. *See* neuron.

bacitracin (*ba-sit-RAY-sin*). Topical antibiotic, applied to the skin to prevent bacterial infection. *See also* antibiotics.

behavioral therapy. Form of psychological treatment sometimes used in the treatment of long-persisting post-herpetic neuralgia (PHN). Behavioral therapy is designed to reduce the effects of pain upon day-to-day behavior, enabling the patient to live a more normal life and to experience pain less intensely.

biofeedback. Electrical amplification of physical signs of psychological stress, sometimes used in the treatment of post-herpetic neuralgia (PHN) to raise awareness of stress and assist relaxation.

booster shot. A dose of vaccine given after initial immunization to maintain or reinforce immunization. *See also* vaccine.

breakthrough infection. Infection that occurs in someone already vaccinated against it. Breakthrough chickenpox infection, after immunization with the varicella vaccine, is uncommon and tends to be relatively mild. *See also* varicella vaccine.

calamine lotion. Anti-itch (antiprurient) medication based on zinc oxide and ferric oxide.

capsaicin (*kap-SAY-ih-sin*). Brand names Zostrix (*ZOS-triks*), Capzacin (*KAP-zah-sin*). Topical medication sometimes used to treat post-herpetic neuralgia (PHN). It is derived from hot peppers, and appears to lower the level of a neurotransmitter that facilitates the passage of pain impulses between neurons (nerve cells). *See also* neurotransmitters.

Capzacin (*KAP-zah-sin*). Brand name for capsaicin.

cataract. Cloudy area in the lens of the eye which may impair vision. Cataracts may result from inflammation of the lens by herpes zoster ophthalmicus. *See also* herpes zoster ophthalmicus.

causalgia (*kaw-ZAL-jah*). Disease that produces burning neurogenic pain in the area of a nerve-damaging injury, such as a severe wound. *See also* neurogenic pain.

chemotherapy. Medical treatment with drugs that kill cancer cells, but that often suppress the immune system as well.

chickenpox. Usually mild, extremely contagious rash disease caused by the varicella zoster virus. Infection results in lasting immunity to chickenpox, but virus surviving in one or more sensory nerve roots may later reactivate, causing shingles.

choroid (*KOR-oid*). Inner lining of the eyeball. The choroid is part of the uvea, a group of connected tissues within the eyeball that can be inflamed and damaged by herpes zoster ophthalmicus. *See also* herpes zoster ophthalmicus, uvea.

ciliary (*SIL-ee-air-ee*) **body**. Part of the uvea, a group of connected tissues within the eyeball that can be inflamed and damaged by herpes zoster ophthalmicus. The ciliary body is a muscular ring connected to the lens by threadlike extensions (cilia), and its main function is to control the focus of the lens. *See also* herpes zoster ophthalmicus, uvea.

cingulum (*SING-yoo-lum*). Latin word from which the name shingles is derived. *Cingulum* means "belt," referring to the typical location of the shingles rash, in a horizontal band around one side of the chest or abdomen. *See also* zoster.

codeine (*KOH-deen*). Narcotic (opioid) occasionally used to relieve the pain of shingles. *See also* narcotics.

cognitive psychotherapy. Type of psychotherapy sometimes used in the treatment of long-persisting post-herpetic neuralgia (PHN). Therapy aims to reconstruct mental attitudes toward pain to encourage coping and healing rather than emotional suffering.

conjunctivitis (*kon-junk-tih-VYE-tis*). Inflammation of the conjunctiva (*kon-junk-TYE-vah*), a transparent mucous membrane that covers and protects the white of the eye. Conjunctivitis is a common complication of herpes zoster ophthalmicus. *See also* herpes zoster ophthalmicus.

controlled breathing. Timed sequence of inhalations and exhalations, used to manage stress through physical relaxation.

cornea (*KOR-nee-ah*). Transparent window of tissue at the front of the eye, through which light passes to the pupil. Inflammation of the cornea (keratitis) caused by herpes zoster ophthalmicus may lead to ulceration or scarring that impairs vision. *See also* herpes zoster ophthalmicus.

corticosteroids (*kor-tih-koh-STER-oidz*). Hormones produced in the outer layer (cortex) of the adrenal glands, or drugs derived from or resembling these hormones. Corticosteroids are often simply called steroids. They relieve the inflammation of shingles, but have some potentially harmful side effects, including the suppression of the immune system.

counterirritation. Mildly irritating sensations that stimulate the central nervous system to inhibit the transmission of more painful sensations. Counterirritants include vigorous massage, rubefacient liniments such as oil of wintergreen, and possibly transcutaneous electrical nerve stimulation (TENS). *See also* rubefacients, transcutaneous electrical nerve stimulation.

cranial (KRAY-*nee-ahl*) **nerves**. Nerves that connect to the brain stem within the skull (the cranium), and that mainly serve the head and neck. *See also* facial nerve, trigeminal nerve.

cytomegalovirus (*sye-toh-meg-ah-loh-VYE-rus*). Herpesvirus that causes a disease with usually mild, flu-like symptoms. If contracted during pregnancy, however, cytomegalovirus can cause birth defects in the baby. *See also* herpesviruses.

cytoplasm (*SYE-toh-pla-zum*). Cell fluid. *See also* neuron.

Darvon (*DAR-von*). Brand name for propoxyphene.

dendrites (*DEN-dryts*). *See* neuron.

dermatome (*DUR-mah-tohm*). Body segment (literally, a "skin slice"), served by one sensory nerve or nerve branch. Shingles is usually confined to a single dermatome.

desipramine (*deh-ZIP-rah-meen*). Brand name Norpramin (*NOR-pra-min*). Tricyclic antidepressant drug used to treat post-herpetic neuralgia (PHN). *See also* antidepressants, tricyclic antidepressants.

diazepam (*dye-AYZ-eh-pam*). Brand name Valium (*VAL-ee-um*). Antianxiety drug that is also prescribed to relieve dizziness caused by shingles of the facial nerve. *See also* Ramsay Hunt syndrome.

DNA. Abbreviation for deoxyribonucleic (*dee-AHK-sih-rye-boh-noo-klee-ik*) acid. Long, twisted, ladderlike molecule known as the double helix, which carries the genetic code for reproduction. Living cells usually contain several strands of DNA, in the form of chromosomes. The varicella zoster virus contains a single DNA molecule, wrapped in a protective coating of protein.

dorsal ganglia (*DOR-sahl GANG-lee-ah*). Enlarged portions of sensory nerve roots, containing the cell bodies of the sensory neurons. The ganglia are located toward the back of the spinal cord (*dorsal* means "back"), near the points where they connect with the central nerves. *See also* peripheral nervous system.

double-blind. Condition required of controlled clinical tests, to eliminate bias and reinforce reliability of results. Subjects are given either the test substance or an inactive placebo, and neither the subjects nor those giving the substances know which is which. *See also* placebo.

EMLA. Abbreviation for eutectic (*yoo-TEK-tik*) mixture of local anesthetics, an ointment containing both lidocaine and prilocaine. *See also* topical anesthetics.

encephalitis (*en-sef-ah-LYE-tis*). Inflammation of the brain and its surrounding membranes, occasionally caused by severe chickenpox or disseminated shingles.

enteric (*EN-tur-ik*) **coating**. Chemical shield that surrounds an oral drug such as aspirin and delays its absorption until it passes through the stomach and reaches the small intestine.

Epstein-Barr virus. Herpesvirus that causes mononucleosis. *See also* herpesviruses.

facial nerve. Composite cranial nerve that has both sensory and motor branches. The sensory branch registers sensations in the area of the ear and the sense of taste in part of the tongue. The motor branch controls facial expressions. Shingles in this and other nearby cranial nerves can cause a condition known as Ramsay Hunt syndrome. *See also* cranial nerves, Ramsay Hunt syndrome.

famciclovir (*fam-SYE-kloh-veer*). Brand name Famvir (*FAM-veer*). Antiviral prodrug, taken orally (by mouth). Prodrugs are chemically converted to active form during absorption into the body. *See also* antiviral drugs, valacyclovir.

gabapentin (*gab-ah-PEN-tin*). Brand name Neurontin (*noo-RON-tin*). Anticonvulsant drug used to treat postherpetic neuralgia (PHN). *See also* anticonvulsants.

ganglia. *See* dorsal ganglia, ventral roots.

glaucoma (*glaw-KOH-mah*). Vision-threatening disease caused by excessive pressure within the eyeball. It sometimes results from the inflammation of herpes zoster ophthalmicus. *See also* herpes zoster ophthalmicus.

guided imagery. Technique for stress management that uses imagination to distract attention away from unpleasant thoughts, feelings, and sensations, including the perception of pain.

herpes simplex, type 1. Herpesvirus that causes oral herpes, or cold sores. *See also* herpesviruses.

herpes simplex, type 2. Virus that causes genital herpes. *See also* herpesviruses.

herpesviruses (*hur-peez-VYE-rus-ez*). A related group of viruses that includes varicella zoster virus, cytomegalovirus, Epstein-Barr virus, and herpes simplex viruses type 1 and type 2. All of them are highly infectious, require a human host, and survive as long as the host does. *See also* virus.

herpes zoster (*HUR-peez ZOS-tur*). Medical name for shingles.

herpes zoster opthalmicus (*ahf-THAL-mih-kus*). Abbreviation HZO. Shingles that originates in the upper, or ophthalmic, branch of the trigeminal nerve of the face. It produces a rash in the area between the forehead and the end of the nose, and often infects the eye. *See also* trigeminal nerve.

HIV. Abbreviation for human immunovirus, a virus that attacks the human immune system and causes AIDS (acquired immune deficiency syndrome).

Hutchinson's sign. Patch of rash near the tip of the nose. It is an early symptom of herpes zoster ophthalmicus, and is considered evidence that the eye will eventually be affected. *See also* herpes zoster ophthalmicus.

hypnosis. Artificially induced state of consciousness (trance) in which the subject becomes strongly susceptible to suggestion. Hypnotism is sometimes used in the treatment of post-herpetic neuralgia (PHN) to distract attention from the perception of pain through such techniques as sensory substitution. *See also* sensory substitution.

HZO. Abbreviation for herpes zoster ophthalmicus.

ibuprofen (*eye-byoo-PROH-fen*). Brand names Advil, Motrin, et al. Widely used over-the-counter nonsteroidal anti-inflammatory drug (NSAID). *See also* nonsteroidal anti-inflammatory drugs.

immune memory. Ability of the immune system to recognize a specific invader, such as a virus, after a first infection.

immune system. System composed mainly of white blood cells and their products which identifies and attacks foreign invaders of the body, such as viruses, bacteria, and funguses.

immunoglobulins. *See* antibodies.

immunosuppressed. Lacking the protection of a normal immune system as the result of aging, disease, genetic defect, drugs, or radiation.

iris. Muscular ring that controls the amount of light passing through the pupil of the eye. The iris is part of the uvea, a group of connected tissues within the eyeball that can be inflamed and damaged by herpes zoster ophthalmicus. Severe inflammation of the iris, called iritis (*eye-RYE-tis*), may lead to vision-threatening glaucoma. *See also* glaucoma, herpes zoster ophthalmicus, uvea.

keratitis (*ker-ah-TYE-tis*). Inflammation of the cornea, a transparent window of tissue at the front of the eye. Keratitis caused by herpes zoster ophthalmicus may lead to ulceration or scarring that impairs vision. *See also* herpes zoster ophthalmicus.

lidocaine (*LYE-doh-kayn*). Topical anesthetic, applied to the skin for temporary relief of pain. *See also* anesthetic.

Lidoderm (*LYE-doh-durm*). Anesthetic patch suffused with lidocaine, used to relieve the pain of post-herpetic neuralgia (PHN). *See also* anesthetic, post-herpetic neuralgia.

Lyrica (*LEER-ih-kah*). Brand name for pregabalin.

malaise. Vague, unspecific sensation of being unwell which is sometimes a preliminary symptom of shingles.

meditation. Technique for stress management which distracts attention away from everyday thoughts, feelings, and sensations, including the perception of pain.

menthol. Topical rubefacient medication. *See* rubefacients.

meperidine (*meh-PER-ih-deen*). Brand name Demerol. Narcotic (opioid) occasionally used to relieve the pain of post-herpetic neuralgia. *See also* narcotics.

MMRV. Abbreviated name for a combination vaccine commonly administered at age twelve months. The initials stand for mumps, measles, rubella (German measles), and varicella (chickenpox). *See also* vaccine.

motor nerves. Peripheral nerves carrying impulses from the central nervous system (brain and spinal cord) to control the movements of muscles. *See also* peripheral nervous system.

Motrin (*MOH-trin*). Brand name for ibuprofen.

naproxen (*nah-PROKS-en*). Brand name Naprocyn (*NAP-roh-sin*). Prescription nonsteroidal anti-inflammatory drug (NSAID). *See also* nonsteroidal anti-inflammatory drugs.

narcotics. Also known as opioids (*OH-pee-oidz*). Pain-relieving drugs either derived from or chemically similar to opium. They inhibit the transmission of pain sensations among nerve cells. Those used to treat shingles are relatively mild forms such as codeine or propoxyphene (Darvon), alone or in combination with other drugs. Stronger forms may be used to treat post-herpetic neuralgia (PHN).

Neosporin (*NEE-oh-spor-in*). Brand name for an ointment combining three antibiotics, applied to the skin to prevent or treat bacterial infection. *See also* antibiotics.

nerve blocks. Techniques to stop the passage of pain sensations through nerves, used occasionally in the treatment of shingles and post-herpetic neuralgia (PHN). Temporary blocks are achieved with injections of local anesthetics. Longer-lasting blocks require severing the nerve by surgery, chemicals, heat, or cold. Blocks may be performed upon sensory nerves, or upon the sympathetic nerves that control autonomic ("self-ruling") body functions. Even long-term blocks produce only temporary relief. *See also* anesthetic, sensory nerves, sympathetic nervous system.

neurogenic (*noor-oh-JEH-nik*) **pain**. Burning or stabbing pain produced by damage or malfunction within neurons (nerve cells). Neurogenic pain is typical not only of shingles, but also of conditions such as trigeminal neuralgia, causalgia, stump pain, and phantom limb pain.

neuron (*NOO-ron*). A single nerve cell. Each neuron of a sensory nerve has a cell body containing the cell nucleus near one end, at the nerve root. From the cell body extends a tubelike axon, ending in branchlike dendrites that receive sensory impulses from the skin and other organs.

Neurontin (*noo-RON-tin*). Brand name for gabapentin.

neurotransmitters (*noor-oh-tranz-MIH-turz*). Chemicals generated by neurons (nerve cells) that pass impulses to other neurons. Several of the drugs used to treat shingles and post-herpetic neuralgia (PHN) either strengthen or inhibit natural neurotransmitters of the nervous system. *See also* anticonvulsants, antidepressants.

nonsteroidal anti-inflammatory drugs. Abbreviation NSAIDs. Drugs such as aspirin and ibuprofen, which relieve the swelling and pain of inflammation. NSAIDs block the production of chcmicals called prostaglandins (*pros-tah-GLAN-dinz*), generated by damaged cells. NSAIDs also affect the perception of pain in the central nervous system.

Norpramin (*NOR-pra-min*). Brand name for desipramine.

nortriptyline (*nor-TRIP-tih-leen*). Brand name Pamelor (*PAM-el-or*). Tricyclic antidepressant drug used to treat post-herpetic neuralgia (PHN). *See also* antidepressants, tricyclic antidepressants.

NSAIDs. Abbreviation for nonsteroidal anti-inflammatory drugs.

oil of wintergreen. *See* rubefacients.

opioids. Medical name for narcotics.

optic nerve. Nerve carrying visual information from the retina of the eye to the brain. The optic nerve can be directly inflamed and damaged by herpes zoster ophthalmicus, or indirectly by glaucoma resulting from the viral infection. *See also* glaucoma, herpes zoster ophthalmicus.

oxycodone (*ok-see-KOH-dohn*). Brand names Percocet (*PUR-koh-set*), Percodan (*PUR-koh-dan*), OxyContin (*ok-see-KON-tin*). Narcotic (opioid) occasionally used to relieve the pain of post-herpetic neuralgia (PHN). *See also* narcotics.

pain clinics. Facilities offering comprehensive, multifaceted treatment of painful disorders such as post-herpetic neuralgia (PHN). Pain clinics employ a team of specialists that may include a neurologist, an anesthesiologist, a physical therapist, and a psychologist, among others.

pain cycle. Condition often resulting from chronic (persistent) pain. Physical pain provokes psychological stress, which in turn intensifies the perception of pain, which leads to more stress, and so on. Even temporary relief from pain may help break the pain cycle.

Pamelor (*PAM-el-or*). Brand name for nortriptyline (*nor-TRIP-tih-leen*), a tricyclic antidepressant drug used to treat post-herpetic neuralgia (PHN). *See also* antidepressants, tricyclic antidepressants.

papules (*PAP-yoolz*). Small bumps that form the first stage of the shingles rash. *See also* pustules, vesicles.

Pepcid (*PEP-sid*). Antiulcer and antiheartburn drug which reduces the production of stomach acid and may counteract the irritation of the stomach lining by nonsteroidal anti-inflammatory drugs (NSAIDs). *See also* nonsteroidal anti-inflammatory drugs.

Percocet, Percodan (*PUR-koh-set, PUR-koh-dan*). Brand names of combination drugs containing oxycodone.

peripheral nerve stimulation. Device implanted under the skin that passes mild pulses of electrical current near a painful sensory nerve, providing pain relief to some patients. *See also* counterirritation.

peripheral nervous system. All the nerves, including the sensory and motor nerves, outside the central nervous system (spinal cord and brain).

phantom limb pain. Neurogenic pain that seems to originate in a limb that has been amputated. *See also* neurogenic pain.

PHN. Abbreviation for post-herpetic neuralgia.

placebo (*plah-SEE-boh*). An inactive substance that resembles the active substance in a double-blind clinical trial. Subjects in the trial may receive either one, and neither they nor those conducting the trial know which is which. Placebo comes from a Latin word meaning "I will please." A placebo may achieve positive results simply because the patient hopes and wishes it to succeed (the placebo effect).

pneumonia. Inflammation of the lungs, occasionally caused by severe chickenpox or disseminated shingles.

post-herpetic neuralgia (*post-hur-PEH-tik noo-RAL-jah*). Abbreviation PHN. Neurogenic pain that persists long after the shingles rash has healed.

pramoxine (*pra-MOK-seen*). Topical anesthetic, applied to the skin for temporary relief of pain. *See also* anesthetic.

prednisone (*PRED-nih-sohn*). Corticosteroid drug, sometimes used to treat shingles. *See also* corticosteroids.

pregabalin (*preh-GAB-ah-lin*). Brand name Lyrica (*LEER-ih-kah*). Anticonvulsant drug used to treat post-herpetic neuralgia (PHN). *See also* anticonvulsants.

prilocaine (*PRIL-oh-kayn*). Topical anesthetic, applied to the skin for temporary relief of pain. *See also* anesthetic.

prodrug. Drug chemically converted to an active form during absorption into the body. *See also* antiviral drugs, famciclovir, valacyclovir.

progressive relaxation. Sequence of exercises to relax muscle groups, one at a time, from the feet to the head. Used for stress management.

propoxyphene (*proh-POK-sih-feen*). Brand name Darvon (*DAR-von*). Narcotic (opioid) occasionally used to relieve the pain of shingles. *See also* narcotics.

prostaglandins (*pros-tah-GLAN-dinz*). Chemicals produced by damaged cells which stimulate pain-sensing nerves. *See also* nonsteroidal anti-inflammatory drugs.

ptosis (*TOH-sis*). Drooping of the upper eyelid. *See also* herpes zoster ophthalmicus.

pustules (*PUS-choolz*). Blisters filled with cloudy pus, which form the third stage of the shingles rash. *See also* papules, vesicles.

Ramsay Hunt syndrome. Group of symptoms caused by shingles of the facial nerve and other nearby cranial nerves. The syndrome may include a rash in and around the ear, severe earache, hearing loss, dizziness, nausea, partial taste loss, and facial muscle paralysis. *See also* facial nerve.

retina. "Screen" at the back of the eye that receives visual images projected through the lens and converts them into sensory impulses to be transmitted through the optic nerve to the brain. The retina can be inflamed and damaged by herpes zoster ophthalmicus. *See also* acute retinal necrosis, herpes zoster ophthalmicus.

rubefacients (*roo-beh-FAY-shents*). "Red-making" liniments and ointments that dilate the blood vessels, causing the skin to flush and feel warm, and also act as counterirritants to the transmission of pain sensations. *See also* counterirritation.

sclera (*SKLAIR-ah*). White of the eye and other outer layers of the eyeball, which may be inflamed by herpes zoster ophthalmicus. *See also* herpes zoster ophthalmicus.

sensory nerves. Peripheral nerves carrying sensory impulses from the skin and other organs to the central nervous system (spinal cord and brain). *See also* motor nerves, neuron, peripheral nervous system.

sensory substitution. Technique for stress management using imagination to substitute a nonpainful sensation, such as coolness or mild prickling, for a painful one.

silver sulfadiazine (*sul-fah-DYE-ah-zeen*). Topical antibacterial drug applied to the skin to prevent bacterial infection.

spinal cord stimulation. Device implanted under the skin that passes mild pulses of electrical current near the spinal root of a painful sensory nerve, providing pain relief to some patients. *See also* counterirritation.

stump pain. Neurogenic pain at the site of an amputation. *See also* neurogenic pain.

sympathetic nervous system. System composed of nerves that control autonomic ("self-ruling") body functions, such as perspiration and blood pressure. Blocking them can sometimes provide temporary relief from neurogenic pain. *See also* neurogenic pain, nerve blocks.

Tagamet (*TAG-ah-met*). Antiulcer and antiheartburn drug which reduces the production of stomach acid and may counteract the irritation of the stomach lining by nonsteroidal anti-inflammatory drugs (NSAIDs). *See also* nonsteroidal anti-inflammatory drugs.

temporal arteritis (*TEM-puh-ral ar-tuh-RYE-tis*). Inflammation of a blood vessel in the temple area of the head, causing pain sometimes mistaken for that of herpes zoster ophthalmicus. *See also* herpes zoster ophthalmicus.

TENS. Abbreviation for transcutaneous electrical nerve stimulation.

topical anesthetics. Medications applied to the skin which not only relieve pain but blunt all sensations, producing temporary numbness. *See also* anesthetic.

topical antibiotics and antibacterials. Medications applied to the skin to prevent bacterial infection. *See also* antibiotics.

topical medications. Lotions, creams, ointments, etc., applied to the skin in order to relieve pain or itching, prevent infection, etc.

tramadol (*TRAM-ah-dol*). Brand name Ultram (*UL-trahm*). Non-opioid painkiller that appears to be effective in relieving the pain of shingles and post-herpetic neuralgia (PHN).

transcutaneous (*tranz-kyoo-TAY-nee-us*) **electrical nerve stimulation**. Abbreviation TENS. Machine that passes mild pulses of electrical current through areas of the skin, providing pain relief to some patients. *See also* counterirritation.

tricyclic antidepressants. Class of antidepressant drugs used in the treatment of post-herpetic neuralgia (PHN). *See also* antidepressants.

trigeminal (*try-JEM-ih-nahl*) **nerve**. Cranial nerve with three branches (*trigeminal* means "triplet") which serves one side of the face. *See also* cranial nerves, herpes zoster ophthalmicus.

trigeminal neuralgia (*noo-RAL-jah*). Inflammation of the trigeminal nerve that causes spasms of stabbing facial pain, sometimes mistaken for herpes zoster ophthalmicus. *See also* herpes zoster ophthalmicus, neurogenic pain, trigeminal nerve.

Ultram (*UL-trahm*). Brand name for tramadol.

uvea (*YOO-vee-ah*). Group of connected tissues within the eyeball that can be inflamed and damaged by herpes zoster ophthalmicus. It is composed of the iris, the ciliary body, and the choroid. *See also* choroid, ciliary body, herpes zoster ophthalmicus, iris.

vaccine. Substance used to immunize against a specific disease. The chickenpox and shingles vaccines are based upon the same strain of varicella zoster virus, which has been attenuated (weakened) so that it cannot multiply and cause disease. But when the vaccine is injected into the body, enough of its chemical structure remains for the immune system to identify it and form antibodies against it. *See also* immune system, varicella zoster virus.

valacyclovir (*val-ah-SYE-kloh-veer*). Brand name Valtrex (*VAL-treks*). Antiviral prodrug, taken orally (by mouth). Prodrugs are chemically converted to an active form during absorption into the body. *See also* antiviral drugs.

Valium (*VAL-ee-um*). Brand name for diazepam.

Valtrex (*VAL-treks*). Brand name for valacyclovir.

varicella (*var-ih-SEL-ah*). Medical name for chickenpox.

varicella vaccine. Highly effective and long-lasting vaccine used to immunize against chickenpox. *See also* vaccine.

varicella zoster (*var-ih-SEL-ah ZOS-tur*) **immune globulin**. Abbreviated VZIG. Concentrate of antibodies to the varicella zoster virus, which can be injected into individuals who have recently been exposed to chickenpox and need extra protection against the virus. *See also* antibodies.

varicella zoster virus. Virus of the herpes group, which causes both chickenpox (varicella) and zoster (shingles). *See also* herpesviruses.

Varivax (*VAR-ih-vaks*). Brand name for the varicella vaccine.

ventral roots. Roots of the motor nerves, which connect to the spinal cord toward its front side. *See also* dorsal ganglia, motor nerves, peripheral nervous system.

vesicles (*VES-ih-kulz*). Small, fluid-filled blisters that form the second stage of the shingles rash. *See also* papules, pustules.

virions (*VIR-ee-onz*). Individual particles of viruses. *See also* virus.

virus. Very small microorganism composed of a single piece of either DNA or RNA, surrounded by a protective coating of protein. Reproduces by invading the nucleus of a living cell and taking over its genetic machinery to produce more virus.

VZV. Abbreviation for varicella zoster virus.

Zostavax (*ZOS-tah-vaks*). Brand name for shingles vaccine. *See also* vaccine.

zoster (*ZOS-tur*). Medical name for shingles, from a Greek word meaning "belt," and referring to the typical location of the shingles rash, in a horizontal band around one side of the chest or abdomen. *See also* cingulum.

Zostrix (*ZOS-triks*). Brand name for capsaicin.

Zovirax (*ZOH-vir-aks*). Brand name for acyclovir.

HELPFUL SOURCES

The following organizations can be helpful in providing you with information and often in recommending a physician or other health-care professional. Many can also provide you with free relevant reading material or a catalog of booklets, books, and tapes for purchase.

Academy for Guided Imagery
10780 Santa Monica Boulevard
Suite 290
Los Angeles, CA 90025
Phone: 800-726-2070
Fax: 800-727-2070
www.academyforguidedimagery.com

American Academy of Dermatology
1350 First Street NW
Suite 870
Washington, DC 20005-3305
Phone: 202-842-3555

Toll-free: 888-462-DERM (3376) and
866-503-SKIN (7546)
Fax: 202-842-4355
www.aad.org

American Academy of Family Physicians
11400 Tomahawk Creek Parkway
Leawood, KS 66211-2672
Mailing Address:
PO Box 11210
Shawnee Mission, KS 66207-1210
Phone: 913-906-6000
Toll-free: 800-274-2237
Fax: 913-906-6075
www.aafp.org

American Academy of Neurology
1080 Montreal Avenue
St. Paul, MN 55116
Phone: 651-695-2717
Toll-free: 800-879-1960
Fax: 651-695-2791
www.aan.com

Amerian Academy of Ophthalmology
PO Box 7424
San Francisco, CA 94120-7424
Phone: 415-561-8500
Fax: 415-561-8533
www.aao.org

American Academy of Pediatrics
141 Northwest Point Boulevard
Elk Grove Village, IL 60007-1098

Phone: 847-434-4000
Toll-free: 800-433-9016
Fax: 847-434-8000
www.aap.org

American Chronic Pain Association (ACPA)
PO Box 850
Rocklin, CA 95677-0850
Phone: 800-533-3231
Fax: 916-632-3208
www.theacpa.org

American Pain Foundation
201 North Charles Street
Suite 710
Baltimore, MD 21201-4111
Phone: 888-615-PAIN (7246)
Fax: 410-385-1832
www.painfoundation.org

American Pain Society
4700 West Lake Avenue
Glenview, IL 60025
Phone: 847-375-4715
Fax: 877-734-8758
www.ampainsoc.org

American Psychiatric Association
1000 Wilson Boulevard
Suite 1825
Arlington, VA 22209-3901
Phone: 703-907-7300
Toll-free: 888-357-7924
www.psych.org

American Psychological Association
750 First Street NE
Washington, DC 20002-4242
Phone: 202-336-5500
Toll-free: 800-374-2721
www.apa.org

Association for Applied Psychophysiology and Biofeed-
back
10200 West 44th Avenue
Suite 304
Wheat Ridge, CO 80333
Phone: 303-422-8436
Toll-free: 800-477-8892
Fax: 303-422-8894
www.aapb.org

National Association of Social Workers
750 First Street NE
Suite 700
Washington, DC 20002-4241
Phone: 202-408-8600
Fax: 202-336-8312
www.socialworkers.org

VZV Research Foundation
1202 Lexington Avenue
Suite 204
New York, NY 10028
Phone: 212-222-3390
Fax: 212-222-8627
www.vzvfoundation.org

INDEX